ELEMENTARY ECONOMIC EVALUATION IN HEALTH CARE

Second edition

TOM JEFFERSON
UK Cochrane Centre and Cochrane Vaccines Field, UK

VITTORIO DEMICHELI
University of Pavia, Italy

MIRANDA MUGFORD
University of East Anglia, UK

BMJ

© BMJ Books 1996, 2000
BMJ Books is an imprint of the BMJ Publishing Group
BMA House, Tavistock Square, London WC1H 9JR

www.bmjbooks.com

First published 1996
by the BMJ Publishing Group
Reprinted 1999
Second edition 2000

British Library Cataloguing in Publication Data

A catalogue record for this book is available
from the British Library

ISBN 0 7279 1478 2

Type set by Saxon Graphics, Derby
Printed and bound in Great Britain by J W Arrowsmith Ltd, Bristol

Contents

Preface

After publication of the first edition of our book, we received a number of very helpful comments and suggestions to improve both content and layout of any future editions.

To our amazement and delight, these comments came from countries as far afield as China, Saipan (in the Pacific Ocean) and South Africa.

In writing the second edition, we have tried to incorporate as many of these comments as possible. We have updated the bibliography, inserted a new chapter (Chapter 8) and attempted to give our readers an up to date overview of the changing field of economic evaluation in a format which we hope is compatible with the elementary nature of the book.

To all the persons who sent us comments we give our heartfelt thanks and look forward to receiving more comments on this edition.

We hope that all our readers, past and present, will recognise our efforts in attempting to update and not to change our winning formula.

TOM JEFFERSON
Viareggio, Italy

Preface to the first edition

Political economy should be seen ... not as a thing by itself, but as a fragment of a greater whole; a branch of social philosophy so inter-linked with all the other branches that its conclusions, even in its own peculiar province, are only true conditionally, subject to inter-ference from causes not within its scope.

J. S. MILL 1806–73

Margin, cost-effectiveness, discounting, sensitivity analysis ... these are words which are read and heard with increasing frequency in health care systems around the world. Those who use them appear almost invested by a supernatural power: that of understanding the mysterious discipline of health economics. In reality, although these words have specific meanings, they are as much a part of health economics —a branch of economics that deals with health systems— as words such as hepatosplenomegaly are a part of medicine. To translate them into plain English we need to grasp the concepts of the underlying science. Once these are understood the "mystery" is no longer.

We, as authors, have followed different paths leading to health economics in general and economic evaluation in particular. Two of us (TJ and VD) are population physicians who first became attracted by what appeared to be the "black art" of health economics and then became involved in its practice. We became involved because the logical concepts which stand behind this seemingly incomprehen-sible jargon were explained by our tutor on our MSc course in words that even we could understand. Once these concepts were within our grasp, we started exploring the subject matter, at first with descriptive exercises and, more recently, with slightly more compli-cated studies.

In the last few years we have tried to span the gap, in our view more imaginary than real, between health economics and medicine and its allied professions. In our journey of discovery we have worked with economists who have invariably welcomed us with open arms in their professional organisations and have provided potent stimulus for our research efforts in areas of health economics hitherto little explored. Throughout, we have had a lot of fun and found the experience rewarding.

The third author (MM) graduated in economics before health economics was regarded as a distinct discipline, but at a time when the application of economic methods to public policy decisions was growing fast. After joining the staff of a multidisciplinary health services research unit, it became clear to her that there was a strong division in health care evaluation between evaluation of the effects on health, done by medical, nursing, midwifery and allied health research specialists, estimation of costs for administrative purposes done by health managers and accountants, and estimates of values and wishes of users of health care, which is the province of social scientists of various disciplines. Economic evaluation needs the insights from each of these disciplines, but also requires modifications of the different approaches, which are not always easily accepted. MM has enjoyed filling this intermediary role, and has been privileged to have been invited by many specialist groups in the field of perinatal care to take part as an equal in discussions about practice and evaluation. She has enjoyed the challenge of finding practical methods for economic evaluation which also make the best use of the methods and results of the research of colleagues in other disciplines.

About the book

It is the intention of this book to introduce health care workers, regardless of their discipline, who may want to embark on a journey of discovery to the most basic principles of health economics and to techniques used in the most commonly used branch of it: economic evaluation of health care.

Health economics is a broad discipline which deals with many different aspects of how health care resources are used. This book will concentrate on principles and techniques of economic evaluation which underpin that part of health economics which aims to facilitate decisions about how resources are best used.

The book is divided into three parts. The first two chapters deal with general and basic concepts and are, by the very nature of the subject matter, theoretical. Chapters 3 to 7 contain a practical example of each type of economic study, Chapter 8 contains a demonstration of how an evidence-based economic model can be constructed, while the last chapter, Chapter 9, deals with current issues of interest. There are four appendices in the book. The first one contains information on how to obtain available data on costs and has a list of references on costing methodologies. In the second appendix is a brief description of forms of economic evaluation applied to management, while the third contains an introduction to decision analysis. Lastly, Appendix 4 is a glossary of terms commonly used by economists, together with their explanation.

Here we need to give a word of warning about basic terminology. In the text, we use words such as "cost-effectiveness analysis" to indicate a specific analytic approach and not, as is the norm these days, as a term to indicate all forms of economic evaluation. If one is embarking on the study of a new discipline, one must have few but clear ideas based on scientific rigour. Similarly, every new term introduced in the text is accompanied by a definition. All definitions used in the book are repeated in the glossary for ease of reference.

In the first part of the book we have tried to concentrate on why things are the way they are in health economics, and, in the second part, on how they should be done. Readers should be aware that, in the rapidly developing health economics scene, some concepts or techniques (such as the calculation of productivity losses caused by disease or injury) are controversial. We have not taken sides in any dispute, confining ourselves to draw our readers' attention to it and indicating possible ways around the problem. Throughout the text we try to give common sense solutions to such methodological problems which remain unresolved. Our "common sense" is also based on what we have found to be accepted practice. Equally, we have tried to mark clearly all the technical and moral pitfalls of which we are aware.

In order to simplify the text, we decided early on to avoid some of the more complicated theoretical concepts (while recognising that these do have their place in a fuller understanding of economic logic) and to avoid producing complicated formulae. We have tried to avoid repetition of concepts and terms but sometimes found it inevitable to have more than one bite at particular cherries for the sake of logical progression of the text.

Each of the method chapters (Chapters 3 to 7) contains a description of the methods introduced, and a practical example, and each of these examples is headed by a summary of the setting of the example and the main issues dealt within. At the end of each example we have introduced a table of research steps which has a common framework based on agreed recommendations for economic evaluation in general. The steps in each table are completed as appropriate for each example. Readers should not seek scientific truths in the outcomes of the examples used in the book. Although these are based on real studies, the data, and sometimes conclusions, have been altered for didactic purposes. Similarly, our book is not meant as a textbook, but only as a "primer" based on our knowledge which, we hope, will whet the appetite of our readers. Those who may want to carry out further reading to enlarge their knowledge can consult the bibliography section at the end of each chapter. Additionally, we have contrived the figure of friendly and available economists to help the fictitious characters to carry out their economic studies in our examples. We strongly advise our readers to consult, at the earliest planning stage, all experts (not just economists) in the various disciplines necessary to carry out methodologically sound studies.

We have selected articles or books containing a more in-depth analysis of the issues examined in the chapter, and, to make choice easier, we have inserted a few comments after each citation. Difficult texts are not included in the bibliography as, in our experience, these are not digestible to the beginner and might very well scare the neophyte away. Inevitably, such a selected bibliography reflects our value judgements.

1 About health economics

Health economics is a logical and explicit framework to aid health care workers, decision-makers, governments, or society at large, to make choices on how best to use resources.

Health economics in its broadest sense deals with several different areas of resource allocation such as, firstly, the public/private debate on the best way to finance health care systems (for example, through international comparative studies of expenditure on health care). Secondly, the study of supply of and demand for health care (for example, through the study of health care markets and barriers to access to health care or ways of influencing the demand for and use of health care services by acting on price or by creating incentives for doctors to enhance, for example, vaccine coverage). Thirdly, by valuing health and assessing the relationship between health and its social and economic determinants (for instance by analysing the relationship between health status and income). Fourthly, the discipline is used as an aid to management of health services (for example, by needs assessment—through the use of either the classic epidemiological/descriptive approach, such as the relative weighting to society of different diseases, or through the use of the technique of marginal analysis).

Finally, there is microeconomic evaluation, which is concerned with comparing the resource implications of alternative ways of delivering health care, for example, an assessment of the efficiency of new health technologies such as magnetic resonance imaging (MRI) scans.

The basis and techniques of microeconomic evaluation form the core of this book, but in Appendix 2 we give a brief description of

1

three of the methods based on the principles of economic evaluation used as an aid to management of health services.

The economic principles which underlie economic evaluation techniques will be dealt with starting from the next chapter, while here we shall introduce a few basic tenets of economic logic as well as giving a brief overview of the history of health economics.

Equity

One of the major preoccupations that economists have is that of equitable distribution of health care resources among all strata of society. This notion, called "equity" (or fair shares), originates from the observation that resources are not equally distributed through modern society. If decisions were taken using only an economic perspective, they would probably reflect the current lack of equity and could perpetuate it or make it worse. This would take place in a sector, such as health care, which has been traditionally regarded to be of universal and equal access.

We do not intend discussing equity (in its many forms) further in this book, but readers should beware of using the techniques which we describe without due attention to their impact on the fair distribution of resources for health care.

The importance of economic evaluation

Health care workers in general and doctors in particular take part with increasing frequency in the process of economic evaluation for several reasons.

Firstly, resources dedicated to health care (as those dedicated to other sectors) have increased but are still limited and under increasing pressure. In poor countries this limitation is absolute, as health care uses resources which are then no longer available for nutrition and shelter. Richer countries have more resources, but also have an increasingly higher offer of new technologies—all of which cannot be acquired simultaneously. Additionally, it is often a population's view that nearly all health care needs must be satisfied, no matter what the costs are. This view is often reinforced by the popular press.

Health care workers find themselves with increasing frequency asking which technology should be provided and which should not, and up to what point the need for health care should be met.

- When the many needs to be met have to be defined and we must compare the costs and benefits of each alternative—this is called *Allocative Efficiency* evaluation.

Rarely are such decisions taken on economic grounds only, and choices rarely are made in an "all or nothing" context. Usually we need to decide upon possible expansion or downsizing of currently met needs. Any change in the quantity of resource used will therefore have to be assessed from the current level and additional costs and benefits will necessarily be incremental or marginal.

The *margin* is the incremental variation in resources committed (inputs) that is required to have a corresponding variation in effects (outputs).

Economic logic and medical ethics

A lot has been written, especially in the 1980s, about a seeming conflict between the ethics of the two disciplines. These doubts may have been based on a misunderstanding of what health economics is about. As we have seen, health economics is a logic framework which allows us to reach conclusions about the best way resources can be allocated, i.e. the way in which most people will benefit. We do not believe that any health care worker can have misgivings about this general aim. Our mission, after all, is to promote health and alleviate suffering. Equally, the possible tension with so-called clinical freedom does not appear to be an insoluble one. Clinical freedom is the faculty of choosing the best intervention for a patient, based on one's knowledge. This choice, however, is always tempered by knowledge of what resources are available. For instance, we are unlikely to achieve the complete disappearance of waiting lists for non-emergency hospital admissions such as for hip replacement. Therefore, for patients who require it, reassurance and interim treatment such as pain-killers and physiotherapy are an acceptable alternative (for both patients and doctors) to immediate admission.

As you can see, economic logic fits into reality easily as it is one more tool that health care workers can employ in order to make such decisions, its only difference being that it makes such choices explicit. Most health care workers welcome explicitness in decision-making and this fits in with contemporary trends in open government.

Tensions, however, do exist on how resources are allocated, not so much because of incompatibility between the ethics of two sciences, medicine and economics, but because of tensions between different perspectives within the same science: medicine. We shall tackle this issue in the next chapter.

The expansion and evolution of Health Economics

The first recorded rudimentary economic valuation of life and limb dates back to the end of the seventeenth century, when Sir William Petty estimated the value of a human life to be between £60 and £90. In Victorian times the writings of pioneers of the sanitary movement, such as William Farr (1807–1883), developed the theme of the relationship between economic growth and workers' health. Farr developed an early version of the *human capital* approach to valuation of productivity losses by calculating a person's monetary value as the current value of the person's projected future earnings minus maintenance. This value he used to calculate the rough benefits of health care during the course of epidemics, thereby applying such values to the advocacy of specific policies.

However, during the latter half of the 19th century and the first half of the 20th century, classical economists gave scant attention to the issue of the use of health care resources, and modern health economics began its relatively young life in the 1950s and 1960s. In the 1950s famous American economists, such as Kenneth Arrow and Milton Friedman, started analysing the application of classic economic theory to health care and, in particular, to two possible uses: as an aid to decisions on how to allocate resources and as a vehicle for social reform.

A decade later, the gathering pace of technological development, an ageing population, and other pressures on resources forced the question: "how should we allocate our scarce resources?" to be asked with increasing frequency. The American school of early pioneers such as Klarman, Fein and Rice began publishing descriptive studies called "cost-of-illness" studies dedicated to calculating the burden to society of particular problems (for example, road traffic accidents, mental illness, infectious diseases).

In the 1970s economists began trying to adapt evaluative techniques of classic economics such as *cost-benefit analysis* (CBA) to health care and to incorporate the descriptive element of *cost-of-illness* methodology into the analytical framework of CBA. This decade saw further development of such techniques with the introduction of *cost-effectiveness analysis* (CEA).

The creation in the late 1970s of a single measure of outcome combining quantity and quality of life which reflects people's preferences for health status (the quality-adjusted-life-year or QALY—pronounced "qualy") led to the birth of cost-utility analysis (CUA), a sibling of CEA.

The themes for the 1990s appear to be further development of the CUA design, with different types of utilities being devised, generically known as health-related-quality-of-life measurement (HRQOL), the relationship between efficiency and effectiveness of interventions, especially of new pharmaceutical products, and the ethics of executing and publishing evaluations. Some of these issues will be examined more closely in Chapter 9.

The steady increase in published economic evaluations during the 1980s can be seen in Figure 1.1 which is based on the work of Elixhauser and colleagues who collected and catalogued a large number of evaluations in their database. Our readers will note the relative demise in popularity of CBA to the advantage of CEA. This factor is probably due in part to methodological difficulties that we shall illustrate in Chapter 7.

Interest in CBA has nevertheless been rekindled by the developments in benefit and welfare measurement, such as willingness to pay and conjoint analysis. A reason for this has been the need for evaluations to incorporate outcomes other than health status, and for

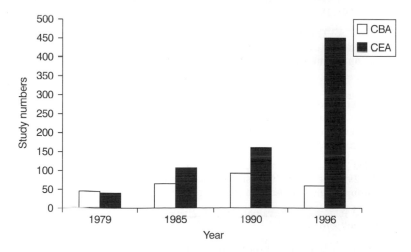

Figure 1.1   *The increase in popularity of economic evaluations (after Elixhauser, 1998)*

evaluation to address broad policy questions beyond those of the health sector.

Suggested reading

Raftery J. Economics notes. Economic evaluation: an introduction. *BMJ* 1998;**316**:1013–14.

(The following series of articles does not attempt a comprehensive description but was intended to discuss issues arising in the design and conduct of economic evaluations.)

Briggs A. Economics notes: handling uncertainty in economic evaluation *BMJ* 1999;**319**:120.

Byford S, Raftery J. Economics notes: perspectives in economic evaluation. *BMJ* 1998;**316**:1529–30.

Palmer S, Byford S, Raftery J. Economics notes: types of economic evaluation. *BMJ* 1999;**318**:1349.

Palmer S, Raftery J. Economics notes: opportunity cost. *BMJ* 1999;**318**:1551–2.

Torgerson DJ, Raftery J Economics notes: measuring outcomes in economic evaluations *BMJ* 1999;**318**:1413 (see also correspondence in *BMJ* **319**:705ff).

Torgerson DJ, Raftery J. Economics notes: discounting. *BMJ* 1999;**319**:914–15.

Williams A. Health economics: the end of clinical freedom? *BMJ* 1988;**297**:1183–6.

Williams A. Cost-effectiveness analysis: is it ethical? *J Med Ethics* 1992;**18**:7–11. (These last two papers represent a clear summary of the relationship between medical ethics and economic logic.)

Elixhauser A, ed. Health care cost-benefit and cost-effectiveness analysis: an update. *Med Care* 1998;3:**361 (supp)**: MJS1–1479. (A database of published economic papers which is a useful starting point for any search, updated to 1996).

Maynard A. Logic in medicine: an economic perspective. *BMJ* 1987;**295**:1541. (The clearest and most concise description of the basis of economic logic that we have come across.)

Robinson R. Economic evaluation in health care. What does it mean? *BMJ* 1993;**307**:670–3.

Robinson R. Economic evaluation in health care. Cost and cost minimization analysis. *BMJ* 1993;**307**:726–8.

Robinson R. Economic evaluation in health care. Cost-effectiveness analysis. *BMJ* 1993;**307**:793–5.

Robinson R. Economic evaluation in health care. Cost-utility analysis. *BMJ* 1993;**307**:859–62.

Robinson R. Economic evaluation in health care. Cost-benefit analysis. *BMJ* 1993;**307**:924–6.

Robinson R. Economic evaluation in health care. The policy context. *BMJ* 1993;**307**:994–6. Very clear introduction to economic evaluation.)

2 The basis of economic evaluation

All of us during our lives would like to conduct more activities and have more interests than we have time and energy to do. In reality, as our resources (for instance, time, skills, and purchasing power) are limited in quantity and availability, we must exercise choice on the way we use what we have. In a similar way, organisations such as hospitals, primary care teams, health departments, and health-purchasing agencies are faced with choices about the best way to use limited resources to achieve their objectives. It was for such purposes that economic evaluation methods evolved.

Resources are scarce not just in a country's economy or in our own purse, but also in health systems and, as a consequence, for those who are served by such systems. No matter how rich and powerful a nation becomes, the amount of resources it devotes to health is, and always will be, limited and in competition with other possible uses.

The economic evaluation approach is followed in commercial investment and option appraisal techniques in which costs and benefits of alternative options are compared. However, where these are based on "market" values of inputs and outputs, they do not take into account the fact that goods and services may be "wrongly" valued from the viewpoint of society. Economic evaluation is of particular importance where prices of goods and services do not reflect the true value of public goods (such as defence, free access to roads, subsidised services), which can only be supplied to everyone, if supplied at all, or are goods and services with no market price (such as voluntary services).

Economic evaluation methods, however, are not meant to substitute the decision-making process or to be the only tool to be

10

used in such a process, which, in any case, is a complex cycle. They are only some of the tools available and are useful in clarifying choices and making such choices explicit. They are used to help us make the best possible use of available resources in a rational decision-making context, when we want to accrue maximum benefits from our scarce resources.

In health care there are many different types of decision to be made. For instance, we may need to decide across many programmes which is the most worthwhile, or which is the best mix of programmes. For example, a health authority may have to decide on whether and at what level to fund teenage health clinics or day centres for the elderly. Alternatively, we may have already decided that something is worth doing and we want to define the best way of achieving it. For example, we will try to prevent an infectious disease by either vaccination or administering γ-globulin.

The conceptual framework of economic evaluation differs according to the type of decisions which it helps to clarify and to the viewpoint of the decision-maker. In the health services, consequences of interventions are numerous and complex. For instance, there are preventive interventions which can avoid the very onset of a disease (for example, polio immunisation), or curative interventions which lengthen survival (cancer treatment), others that modify the quality of survival (pain relief) and others still that modify both (kidney transplants). Some interventions can have negative effects or no effects. Some effects take place on both the patient and his/her family or other patients, or in a more indirect manner on society as a whole, for instance, causing productivity losses through sickness. Again, such losses can accrue to society, to the patient or his/her family, or to carers, and their consequences are taken into account in economic evaluation to allow comparison with inputs, as health economics is a science concerned mainly with the bottom line: the total benefits or damage arising from our actions.

To provide health care interventions or programmes, we need resources. Resources are all that society owns and uses to provide such programmes. The same resources are not available for an alternative use, i.e. they can be used only once. Both tangible items (equipment, premises, drugs, ambulances, materials, money) and intangible items (time, knowledge, and know-how) must be taken into account, regardless of whether they are used by and accrue to health services, society, industry, or the single individual.

11

In order to make comparisons between the options it is necessary to find a common unit of value for each of the inputs, during and as a consequence of the health care intervention. If it is relevant for the type of evaluation being conducted, the health consequences are also valued in common units.

Complete economic evaluations aim to clarify, quantify and value all the relevant options, and their inputs and consequences. Cost-benefit analysis (CBA) falls into this category. Some approaches fall short of full valuation of all consequences, but are still considered to be economic evaluations. This includes most cost-utility analyses (CUA), cost-effectiveness analyses (CEA) and cost-minimisation analyses (CMA).

Many studies of use of resources in health care do not make explicit comparisons between options for care. These are not economic evaluations, but nevertheless can be considered as economic studies and can contribute to our understanding. For this reason we have included a description of cost-of-illness (COI) methods in this book.

Methods of economic evaluation

/All methods of economic evaluation have one principle in common: they examine one (or more) possible interventions and compare the inputs or resources necessary to carry out such interventions with their consequences or effects/

The various methods of economic evaluation differ in the way they itemise and value inputs and consequences. Such differences reflect different aims and viewpoints of the decision-making problems.

Cost-minimisation analysis (CMA)—when the consequences of the intervention are the same, then only inputs are taken into consideration. The aim is to decide the cheapest way of achieving the same outcome.

Cost-effectiveness analysis (CEA)—when the consequences of different interventions may vary but can be measured in identical natural units, then inputs are costed. Competing interventions are compared in terms of cost per unit of consequence.

Cost-utility analysis (CUA)—when interventions which we compare produce different consequences in terms of both quantity and quality of life, we express them in utilities. These are measures which comprise both length of life and subjective levels of well-being (the best known utility measure is the quality-adjusted-life-years or QALYs). In this case, competing interventions are compared in terms of cost per utility (cost-per-QALY).

Cost-benefit analysis (CBA)—when both the inputs and consequences of different interventions are expressed in monetary units so that they compare directly and across programmes even outside health care.

All methods of economic evaluation value inputs and consequences following the same three-stop road. Firstly we must identify inputs and consequences, secondly they must be measured using appropriate physical units, and lastly we must value them.

Problems are encountered in all three phases. Some items are difficult to identify as some health care interventions have hidden or unknown costs and consequences. Not all costs and consequences can be measured in appropriate physical units as some interventions have intangible consequences, such as the reduction of pain or the increase in the quality of one's social performance. Other programmes use inputs which are equally difficult to quantify, such as hi-tech know-how.

Values of resources are assigned by defining costs. These are considered by economists to be the benefits of opportunities foregone, i.e. the best possible alternative use of the same resources (opportunity cost). Such a definition of cost carries several implications. Firstly, costs do not equate with expenditure, as all that can be used in an alternative manner is a cost, even though it appears freely available and there does not appear to be a market for it (such as fresh air, or a voluntary worker's time). Secondly, values, and hence costs, vary according to value judgements and other factors (such as timespan) which depend on individuals, society, scarcity, and need. Valuing inputs and consequences is the most difficult aspect of conducting an economic evaluation as, in reality, the only readily available measures of value, prices, exist only where there are true markets, and these cover only a minority of health inputs and consequences. The problems relating to valuing such "missing" items will be examined in the following chapters.

Inputs and consequences of a health intervention accrue at different times, especially for chronic diseases and the population-based programmes to deal with them. In this case we cannot directly compare the inputs of a programme starting today with its consequences which will accrue in 30 years' time. So economists "bring forward" the value of such consequences by using a technique called *discounting* which allows the calculation of the present values of inputs and benefits which accrue in the future. Discounting is based mainly on a time preference which assumes that individuals prefer to forego a part of the benefits if they accrue it now, rather than fully in the uncertain future. The strength of this preference is expressed by the discount rate which is inserted in economic evaluations. The choice of a discount rate and the choice of which items it should be applied to are a matter of intense debate among economists.

The comparison between inputs and consequences does not happen in a vacuum, its context influences the comparison itself. For instance, production costs are dependent on numbers of units produced. For example, as production rises, costs may decrease if fixed costs (those that do not vary with the production) are divided by a larger number of units and no other investment is necessary. Often the choice is not about whether to carry out a certain intervention or not but about varying the volume of services currently provided or shifting resources between services. The comparison then must be based on inputs necessary at that level of variation and the change in consequences that results from that variation of inputs. This type of logic is called *marginal* and is at the basis of all the costing procedures which economists use. All comparisons made within the framework of an economic evaluation are based on marginal logic.

Evaluations are models which attempt to capture and summarise reality. However, the effects of health care are often uncertain and our models tend to be based on real data (epidemiological, clinical, or resource data) which are often either incomplete or of dubious quality, or are simply not there. Epidemiology, for instance, provides us with an estimate of probabilities (of developing a particular disease, or of effecting a transition from one stage of the disease to the next), or even a range of estimates which is at times wide. Where data are absent or uncertain, the gap may have to be filled by assumptions. In order to deal with uncertainty and carry on with our decision-making process, economic evaluations use a range of techniques, called *sensitivity analysis*, which repeats the comparison between inputs and consequences varying the assumptions underlying the estimates. In other words it tests the robustness of the conclusions by varying the items around which there is uncertainty.

In the following chapters we clarify and further explore the issues just outlined. They are further detailed using various examples which illustrate the strengths and weaknesses of each design and which explain the practical application of these concepts. We start with the description of the economic impact of asthma through the means of COI methodology (Chapter 3) and we then look at our first economic evaluation design (CMA) by comparing the cheapest way to achieve BP control (Chapter 4). In Chapter 5 we introduce CEA design and the use of sensitivity analysis by assessing the cheapest way to avoid post-caesarean section wound infection, while in Chapter 6 we introduce health state valuation within the framework of CUA. Chapter 7 contains an example of a CBA to aid a decision on whether or not to vaccinate a whole population, together with further valuation methodology and an application of discounting.

At the end of the methodological chapters (3–7) we summarise the important steps in the conduct of the studies, highlighting how these were applied in each study, when relevant. An outline of these steps is listed in Box 2.1.

In Chapter 8 we discuss the problem of using economic evaluations in practical decision making with a scenario. In this case, however, methods are not so well understood or developed.

Box 2.1   Research steps for economic evaluation

- Specification of the question, and baseline comparison group
- Specification of the viewpoint, type and coverage of economic study
- Specification of key outcome and estimation of effectiveness
- Specification of method for valuation of health outcomes
- Definition of costs to be estimated
- Estimation of differences in quantities of resource use
- Estimation of unit costs of elements of resource use
- Specification of analytic model
- Taking account of time preference
- Summarise economic result
- Sensitivity analysis

Suggested reading

Drummond MF. *Studies in economic appraisal in health care*. Oxford: Oxford University Press, 1981.

Drummond MF, Ludbrook A, Lowson K, Steele A. *Studies in economic appraisal in health care*, vol 2. Oxford: Oxford University Press, 1986. (Critical appraisals of published economic evaluations. It is very helpful to see these clearly laid out examples in deciding whether and how to adopt a particular method or approach.)

Drummond MF, O'Brien B, Stoddart GL. *Methods for the economic evaluation of health care programmes*. 2nd edition. Oxford: Oxford University Press, 1997. (A user-friendly textbook which has been read by generations of students of economic evaluation.)

HM Treasury. *Economic appraisal in central government: a technical guide for government departments*. London: HMSO, 1991. (A guide to appraisal of projects or programmes for public spending, presenting an official view about appropriate assumptions, methods and sources for studies to inform government spending priorities.)

Williams A. The cost-benefit approach. *Br Med Bull* 1974;**30**:252–6. (A classic rallying call to the cause, giving justification for economic evaluation and pointing out the unethical aspect of decision making without considering economic issues.)

3 Cost-of-illness studies (COI)

Cost-of-illness (COI) studies, sometimes also known as burden-of-illness studies, were among the first economic studies to appear in the literature. The first COI study mentioned in modern bibliographies dates back to 1920. In the late 1950s and early 1960s COI studies became increasingly popular.

The aim of COI studies is descriptive: to itemise, value, and sum the costs of a particular problem with the aim of giving an idea of its economic burden. Traditionally, COI studies have been used to highlight and to weight different health problems for comparative purposes, both within a national context and internationally. In a traditional Public Health approach, health problems are usually weighed by expressing their measures of occurrence (incidence and prevalence), seriousness (mortality), and overall weight (costs). Although COI studies are not complete economic evaluations, their aim is still to inform choices in resource allocation by estimating resource consequences of health problems in relation to each other.

Describing the social weight of an illness, and the definition of its place among other illnesses, not only heightens awareness of the problem but aids its insertion in a list of priorities. Thus, COI studies can help to focus society's attention on health and assist the decision-making process. Because they are studies of resource use and aim to affect the debate on allocation of resources, COI fall within the field of economics. More recently COI studies have increased in frequency as the pharmaceutical industry seeks to establish the worthiness of illnesses as commercial targets. Some COI studies are also used as precursors to full economic evaluations of the introduction of drugs or appliances, as the methods of valuing consequences are at times the same in both evaluations and COI studies. COI methodology, also used in the UK by research planning and commissioning groups, has been criticised because it takes into account only the costs of resources but not of the utility gain of reducing the illness. COI studies also do not compare alternative uses of resources and therefore may not adequately measure opportunity costs.

The essence of the methods employed in COI studies is:

• recognition
• identification
• listing
• measurement and
• valuation

of costs generated by an illness. These stages are common to costing methodology used in all evaluations, no matter how complex. However, such a methodology is only applied here to consequences and not to inputs. In this chapter we shall use the term "costs" to indicate the burden of an illness, and we will confine the use of the term "consequences" to the following chapters where interventions and their consequences are evaluated. Readers can consult Appendix 1 of this book for a list of recommended references to costing methodology and a list of sources of cost data.

The first stage of the COI methodology is the identification of all cases of the illness in question; usually this is done on the basis of national statistics, if available, or by extrapolating to the whole population from a smaller survey. This stage suffers from the limitations of the epidemiological data on which it is based, such as difficulty in case definition, incomplete knowledge of the natural history of the disease, under-notification of cases, and so on.

The second stage consists of identifying the costs generated by all the cases of the illness. Identification can be aided by a systematic qualitative research approach to identify all points of view of interested parties.

Traditionally, COI studies have examined the following costs:

Direct costs—borne by the health care system, community and family in directly addressing the problem.

Indirect costs—mainly productivity losses caused by the problem or diseases, borne by the individual, family, society, or by the employer.

Intangible costs—usually the costs of pain, grief and suffering and loss of leisure time. The cost of a life is usually included in case of death.

Rarely are such costs calculated for all cases of the illness identified in the study, especially if this is a national one. More often a sample of cases is costed and the results are extrapolated to the population of cases.

Two alternative strategies are used to collect cost data: the incidence and the prevalence strategies. The former approach costs cases from their onset to their disappearance for whatever reason (usually cure or death), while the latter costs all cases in a short period irrespective of the stage they are at. The incidence strategy is more precise but is usually used only for those diseases which have short duration (i.e. infectious diseases). The prevalence strategy relies on more assumptions, but is often the only practicable way to cost chronic diseases.

In general, COI studies are concerned with defining the value of resources directly used up by the illness and not their overall cost. For example, one of the possible resource items of an illness is the number of days in hospital because of that illness. The total cost of such a hospital stay, however, does not represent the real "burden" of the illness to society as a part of the hospital costs are fixed and are independent from the existence of the disease. To identify the value of the resources directly used by the cases of the illness, COI studies estimate the "avoidable costs". These are the costs which are generated by the illness and which would be avoided if the illness did not occur. Avoidable costs are only gross estimates of values and seem inadequate, particularly to value indirect and intangible costs. Even so, the calculation is far from straightforward, and how to establish the avoidable costs of resources such as GP's time, preventive measures, and so on, is currently a matter of continuing debate.

The alternative manner of assessing values could be the so-called "willingness to pay" (WTP) approach, which sizes the burden of a disease by measuring what society would be prepared to pay in order to avoid that disease or problem. The concept is appealing because both opportunities and values are simultaneously considered but the practical application of WTP is full of difficulties, relating mainly to the questions asked and the meaning of answers given. Whereas the usual viewpoint for COI studies is the societal one, estimates of WTP are derivable only from individuals. It is unlikely that individuals have enough information to weigh up the value to themselves of avoiding the disease, and they certainly do not have the information to assess the same value to society (see Chapter 7).

19

COI studies are interested in values, but deriving them is still problematic, this being a problem in common with most forms of economic evaluation. A sizeable number of COI studies, especially in the past, simply did not tackle the problem and presented lists of resources costed through their average costs leading often to unreliable and over-inflated assessments of the burden of diseases.

Scenario for cost-of-illness study

A description of the social burden of acute asthma in a local community, based on the gathering of one calendar year's data, the so-called incidence approach. The study takes into account the different use of services for asthma, and its main motivation is an attempt at highlighting the importance of acute asthma as a health problem.

Dr Black is a university lecturer working on the development of a drug to prevent acute asthma. His biggest problem is to obtain funding for his idea. He decides he will try to demonstrate the burden of illness that his drug would remove, if successful. He wants to convince his potential backers that even a large outlay would be worthwhile in terms of morbidity prevented. He teams up with Dr Cutts, a hospital physician with a special interest in acute asthma. Dr Cutts is trying to raise the profile of acute asthma. Their first idea is to master the COI technique to demonstrate the economic burden of acute asthma. As Cutts' hospital firm is the only one in the radius of 80 kilometres specialising in respiratory medicine, they decide to estimate the costs of all cases in the catchment area.

Black and Cutts set their aim: to describe the cost of acute asthma in that community. They decide that they will adopt the viewpoint of society and calculate both direct and indirect costs of hospital treatment. As asthma is an acute and reversible disease, they decide to look at one year's costs only. This viewpoint will dictate both the type of costs and cost components taken into consideration. As this is their first study, Black and Cutts ask an economist friend of theirs, Dr Stones, for advice throughout the study.

The first step they take is the identification of all acute asthma cases, getting an idea of how many cases are seen each year, their age and severity mix to calculate how many resources they use up. Black and Cutts opt for a case definition for acute asthma based on ICD 9 493 (episodic wheezing). To check the accuracy of hospital coding they take the names of the last ten patients seen on the wards and match them with the hospital record system.

As acute asthma is relatively short-lived, Stones suggests that the incidence strategy would be the best. However, as they start in May 1996, if they were to base their calculations on an exclusively prospective data collection exercise, this would mean either losing all seasonal cases or waiting a longer time for the answer. Black and Cutts decide to go for a cohort study design with a mixed retrospective-prospective cohort study design. The retrospective phase will gather data on asthma cases back to the beginning of the year and the prospective exercise will gather data from the day of the start of collection to the end of the year.

Black and Cutts decide that they will initially calculate a cost per episode so that at a later date they can model total economic burden by different incidence rates of acute asthma. Later this would enable them to answer questions such as: "how much would asthma cost in your community if the incidence were 50% lower than the present one?".

Next, they devise a data collection proforma which will enable them to itemise, measure, and value resources used by acute asthmatics. Stones advises them that the easiest way of conceptualising the task is to follow (on paper) each acute asthma patient through an "episode of care", carefully recording the amount of resources consumed. Cutts examines what COI literature he has available in search of inspiration and finds several good examples, based mainly on communicable diseases.

Black and Cutts have a go at describing all possible direct costs generated by acute asthma cases in their hospital. However, as their aim is to estimate the cost of acute asthma both in hospital and the community for the year 1996, they must take into consideration the likely extra-hospital resources used up by acute asthmatics. They conduct a qualitative survey, speaking with patients, their families, and all health care workers involved to identify all possible costs generated by asthma and all possible viewpoints. They decide to measure the quantity of each resource item and then multiply it by its unit cost to achieve a total cost. Each resource must be measured in its appropriate unit and their resource worksheet looks like that in Table 3.1.

Their list is probably too long, but as this is their first COI study they do not want to omit any item. Black and Cutts realise that some of the resources were measured in a possibly controversial manner. For example, the measurement of hospital length of stay in days may not take account of the fact that the first days after admission are the

Table 3.1   The resource measurement worksheet for Drs Black, Cutts and Stones' COI study

Resource	Quantity
Direct costs	
Hospital (hotel care)	Days
Specialised care (intensive care)	Days
Nursing staff	Hours
Medical staff	Hours
Treatment (including consumables)	Number of each item
Investigations	Number of each item
Hospital overheads	Apportioned on the basis of time spent in the hospital
General practitioner contacts	Number
Community nurse visits	Number
Drugs	Number of each item
Investigations	Number of each item
Indirect costs	
Patient and family	
Travel costs (hospital or clinic)	Kilometres
Informal support	Hours
Other expenses (remedies, diet, air humidifier etc.)	Acquisition costs

ones that cost most. They decide, however, to use those measures which are available and are reasonably valid for their hospital in that setting. For instance, they know that length of stay for asthma has little variability and purchasers do not pay out a different amount for the first and last days.

Black and Cutts now add indirect costs to the bill, although they have heard that methods for estimation are shrouded in controversy. Black and Cutts are well aware that asthma has multiple influences on all sectors of society and, without doubt, sickness absence, because the disease causes economic loss which must be taken into account when calculating the total burden of disease. As they are uneasy at costing intangibles, they decide to limit their calculations to tangible costs only (the problems linked with the calculation of intangible costs will be further addressed in Chapter 7). The following item is added to the list: days off work or school because of acute asthma.

Cutts and Black decide that they are unable to value intangibles but are aware that Ms Webb, a behavioural scientist in the same region, has been carrying out an in-depth qualitative observational study of psychological health and social conditions of life for asthma sufferers. This study, sponsored by the Health Education Authority, who have been contracted to implement an asthma self-management campaign, is not yet completed. They may at a later stage add information from this study to their report.

Next comes the problem of defining the unit costs of resource items. Starting from the hospital, they discover that although they had listed more than one type of hospital resource, there is the possibility to calculate a unit cost per case of asthma without having to add up the single components. This is due to the fact that Cutts' hospital has an extensive DRG-based accounting system. Calculated costs are specific to these patients and comprise their share of hospital overheads. DRGs, or diagnostic-related groups, are means of classifying patients by the same amount of resources consumed (so called "isoresource"), irrespective of pathology.

DRG-based costs, however, are average and this will entail further refinement at the valuation stage. Dr Stones advises them that DRG costs reflect input costs and do not match the hospital price list, which is based on charges.

For GP cost items they decide to use average yearly pay figures, divided by the total number of patient contacts made. For nurse visits they derive hourly pay gross rates. For drugs they use acquisition prices, whereas for investigations they use the local private clinic tariff. To estimate the unit cost of one kilometre they use the National Health Service official rate. Informal care unit costs are derived from market prices for home-helps, whereas remedies and appliances are costed at acquisition price.

Productivity losses are costed by deriving daily gross rates of pay for the affected individual or his or her family. This theoretically represents the unit of loss due to asthma for that person.

Now Black and Cutts proudly display their work to their friend Stones. He warns them that they require one more step to complete the exercise: that of valuation of the costs arising from the disease. The value of the benefits foregone because of the disease might be estimated by the willingness of a representative sample of the population to pay to avoid the disease (the WTP approach—see Chapter 7). The alternative method, more in tune with the approach that Black and Cutts had followed, is to value the benefits foregone by the resources used as a consequence of the disease (opportunity cost approach).

They go for the latter approach, although this cannot be applied to all items. For some they will just have to assume an avoidable element. Black and Cutts start by agreeing that at least 80% of

23

hospital costs are unavoidable as they are fixed and are due mainly to staff costs. As asthma accounts for a minor proportion of admissions, it is unlikely that its disappearance would cause a sizeable drop in costs. On Stones' advice they reduce the DRG-based unit cost by 80%. As the cost of GPs' contracts is calculated on a capitation basis and the cost is small, its avoidable fraction is likely to be so small as to be not worth including.

Nurses in that district are very busy, so Black and Cutts decide that the avoidable fraction is as high as their hourly wage. They apply the same reasoning to drugs and investigations, transport costs, informal support, and other expenses. They decide to calculate productivity losses only for losses which actually occurred. For instance, one of the patients is a barber who had to close his shop for the 3 days of his admission and 2 days of recovery, thereby losing income. Similarly, other patients had sick pay instead of their full entitlement. They add the item "real loss of income" to the list.

According to the registers of the clinic, 100 patients were admitted with acute asthma to the ward in 1995. It seems reasonable to assume that between 90 and 110 would be admitted in 1996. A few more in the community would probably not be admitted or go elsewhere. Black and Cutts calculate that it will require 1 hour per case to elicit or retrieve the information required on the proforma. As there are no funds, they each schedule 50 hours for data collection and loading.

As Black and Cutts start their data collection, going through hospital records and recording new data prospectively, they also start building an epidemiological map of the problem. They discover that, in the first 4 months of 1996, there were 42 admissions for acute asthma, of which 10 were re-admissions. They decide to give each case a study number and to keep a separate tally of the re-admissions (defined as those re-admitted within 1 week of discharge), prefixing their study number with the letter "R". Such a precaution is taken because Cutts knows that re-admissions have a different set of admission tests from the others, in other words their resource consumption pattern is likely to be different. They also decide to calculate an age-specific breakdown as they realise that consumption of certain items varies with age. At the end of the year their epidemiological model looks like the one in Table 3.2. Thankfully there have been no deaths.

The data collection proforma is structured around the list of resources consumed by each case. Each patient record is identified by a study number. Cutts holds the key to both study and hospital

Table 3.2   Drs Black, Cutts and Stones' epidemiological model for their COI study

	Age			
	0–14	15–64	65+	Total
All admissions	65	23	17	105
First admissions	45	22	13	80
Subsequent admissions	20	1	4	25
Casualty contacts	73	27	28	128

records. Hence, if required, more data are available while confidentiality is preserved.

Next comes the problem of ascertaining whether the cases described are an underestimation of the total acute asthma cases in the territory for 1996 and, if so, by how much. From the literature they derive a general admission rate for acute asthma. Applied to their catchment area, this indicates that up to 30 cases may have been missed. They decide to include the costs of these patients as "community cases", i.e. without hospital costs. Having collected the data and calculated the costs and values per patient they derive the final table based on all ages and only on hospital admissions (Table 3.3).

Table 3.3   Drs Black, Cutts and Stones' cost calculations for their COI study (1996 prices)

Resource	Quantity		Unit costs (£, 1996)	Total costs		Avoidable fraction	
	min	max		min	max	min	max
Direct costs							
Hospital (days)	0	1.5	130	0	19.5	0	38.2
GP contacts	1.7	2.5	10	17	25	—	—
Nurse hours	0	1.6	8	0	13	0	13
Drugs							
Bronchodilators	0.8	3.6	6	4.8	21.6	4.8	21.6
Other	0	1.1	6	0	6.6	0	6.6
Investigations							
Lung function tests	0.9	1.4	3	2.7	4.2	2.5	3.8
Other	0	1.9	9	0	17.1	0	17.1
Indirect costs							
Patient and family							
Travel costs (km)	2.9	3.9	0.10	0.3	0.4	0.3	0.4
Informal support (hour)	0	1.3	5	0	6.5	0	6.5
Other expenses	—	—	—	—	—	—	—
Days off work (days)[a]	1.7	2.4	21	35.7	50.4	0	5[a]
Total				61	340	7.6	105.6

[a]The avoidable fraction of days off work is the mean of the whole real productivity losses sustained.

Now Dr Black wants to extrapolate the results to the whole UK population. Stones points out that this should be properly done on the basis of age-specific and admission and re-admission-specific avoidable costs. Black and Cutts go back to their database and calculate the table for each group.

Our researchers have now completed their estimates which show an avoidable cost per case of about £1002.14.

Conclusion

Several assumptions went into our exercise. First of all, readers' familiarity with cohort study design. The more experienced will know that the retrospective phase of data collection is likely to yield a few problems, as not all the kinds of data that our friends want are likely to have been recorded on patients' notes and, if they are, they may be in a different format. This problem always leads the researcher to try to either fill in the gaps or guess.

What do the data tell us? Although the usefulness of such data is limited, as there is no comparator available, Black still has a good weapon as the global incidence of the disease is higher than the resource he needs to develop his idea. Research backers may or may not be impressed by this type of exercise, and a lot will depend on the effectiveness of Black's idea. You will be glad to know that Black has sent a copy of his proposal with a copy of the study to the Department of Health and has been asked to submit a full proposal for the research.

Dr Cutts has discovered that there is a very high consumption of bronchodilators in his firm. He has now set up a group to draw some guidelines and wants to reduce consumption by 25%.

Areas of controversy

Few economists consider COI studies as real economic evaluations as they do not define choices and do not directly help in making them. Additionally, COI studies have in the past been conducted with dubious methods. Over-reliance on average costs rather than marginal ones has led in some cases to a systematic overestimation of the burden of the problem. Additionally, methods for estimation of indirect costs are the subject of discussion. In this chapter we will deal with the tangible cost controversy only (see also Chapter 7).

Nobody doubts that productivity losses due to disease actually take place, but the problem has centred on how to value them. The traditional method has always been that based on the human capital concept, whereby production losses due to disease are estimated by summing the wages of the individuals affected (very much like Black and Cutts have done). Recently, such a method has drawn the criticism of those, like Koopmanschap and Rutten, who believe that for short-term absence, somebody's work can be covered by a colleague, whereas in the long term an unemployed person can be hired (especially in countries of high unemployment). The majority of the economic loss falls on the sick person, and on his or her employer, but not on society—hence the importance of presenting costs separated from resources. They propose the use of the so-called "friction method" which relies on local knowledge of the employment market and which leads to lower estimates than the human capital method. Such a controversy is not trivial given that, as in our example, indirect costs form a large part of economic losses.

Finally, COI studies rely on a reasonable knowledge of the epidemiology of a problem. Frequently in practice, however, uncertainties about the real number of cases and transition probabilities between disease stages are added to economic methodology uncertainties, limiting the power of such studies.

Despite these caveats, the methods adopted by Black and Cutts are reasonable, provided that the assumptions made and the reasoning behind them are made clear in the text. With an increasing momentum towards disclosure of detailed methodology used in all studies, when the aim of the exercise is to publish, authors should keep their data and calculations handy as referees may want to scrutinise them.

An evolution of the classic epidemiological approach to COI estimation is WHO's global burden of disease (GBD). In the GBD study the burden of disease is calculated by length of life weighted by the disability due to a specific disease. The synthetic measure is called disability adjusted life year (DALY). Since their introduction in 1996, DALYs have attracted considerable interest and criticism. They have the undoubted merit, however, of being a potential measure of burden and outcome.

COI studies are a good training ground for budding economic evaluators as description of a problem always precedes its analysis. Readers should not be discouraged by controversy and should bear in mind that most economists undertake COI studies routinely.

The golden rule is:

- Keep direct and indirect costs separate and show resources and unit costs in different columns
- Do not assume that you have identified all the relevant costs and benefits.

Suggested reading

Drummond MF. Cost-of-illness studies. A major headache? *PharmacoEconomics* 1992;2:1–4. (A good résumé of the controversy on the role of COI studies.)

Drummond MF, McGuire AJ, Black NA, Pettigrew M, McPherson CK. Economic burden of treated benign prostate hyperplasia in the UK. *Br J Urol* 1993;**71**:290–6. (A good quality COI study.)

Harrington W, Krupnick AJ, Spofford WO. *Economics and episodic disease. The benefits of preventing a giardiasis outbreak.* Washington, DC: Resources for the future, 1991. (A very detailed COI study of an outbreak of *Giardia lamblia* with exhaustive questionnaire examples.)

Koopmanschap MA, Rutten FFH. Indirect costs in economic studies: confronting the confusion. *PharmacoEconomics* 1993;**4**:446–54. (A summary of the indirect cost valuation controversy.)

Murray CJL, Lopez AD. Mortality by cause for eight regions of the world. Global burden of disease study. *Lancet*; **349**: 1269–76.

Murray CJL, Lopez AD. Regional pattern of disability—free life expectancy and disability-adjusted life expectancy. Global burden of disease study. *Lancet*;**349**:1347–52.

Murray CJL, Lopez AD. Global mortality, disability, and the contribution of risk factors. Global burden of disease study. *Lancet*;**349**:1436–42.

Murray CJL, Lopez AD. Alternative projections of morbidity and disability by cause 1990–2020. Global burden of disease study. *Lancet*; **349**:1498–1504.

Rice DP. Cost-of-illness studies: fact or fiction? *Lancet* 1994;**344**:1519. (One-page summary from the doyenne of COI.)

Roberts JA, Sockett PN. The socio-economic impact of human *Salmonella enteritidis* infection. *Int J Food Microbiol* 1994;**21**:117–29. (A good quality COI study.)

Rutten-van Molken MPM, van Doorslaer EKA, Rutten FHF. Economic appraisal of asthma and COPD care: a literature review 1980–91. *Soc Sci Med* 1992;**35**:161–75. (Review of the economics of asthma.)

Research steps for a cost-of-illness study

Stage of economic evaluation	Example
Specification of the question, and baseline comparison group	Estimating the costs of asthma in a community, no comparison group
Specification of the viewpoint, type and coverage of economic study	Societal viewpoint. Cost of illness study, costs for one year
Specification of key outcome and estimation of effectiveness	Not relevant in COI
Specification of method for valuation of health outcomes	Not relevant in COI
Definition of costs to be estimated	Direct costs include hospital and primary care, and patients' travel. Indirect costs include days off work
Estimation of differences in quantities of resource use	Analysis of hospital and primary care records provided estimates of use of health services. Patient interviews used to estimate time lost from work
Estimation of unit costs of elements of resource use	Hospital DRG data, national average pay rates for health care labour and valuation of day off work, acquisition prices for drugs and tests
Specification of analytic model	Simple cumulation of costs per case. Estimation of "avoidable" costs from prevention of disease
Taking account of time preference	Not applicable in this short term COI
Summarise economic result	Cost per case
Sensitivity analysis	Not done in this example

4 Cost-minimisation analysis (CMA)

As we have seen, economic evaluation models are based on the analysis of the relationship between inputs, which are usually different one from another, and their consequences. Such as analysis has the aim of identifying the most efficient intervention, i.e. that which makes best use of scarce available resources. If health care interventions which are assessed by economic evaluation have the same qualitative and quantitative consequences, then economic analysis can concentrate on inputs, and disregard consequences. This is the case in cost-minimisation analysis (CMA), which we will examine in this chapter.

The nub of the design of CMA is the identification of the intervention with the lowest possible costs. Despite this conceptual simplicity, there are aspects of the method which need to be carefully considered. First of all, we must be absolutely sure that the consequences are the same. All health care interventions have multiple impacts on one or more dimensions (social sphere, physical and psychological well-being) and some of these may not be obvious.

Secondly, not only must such consequences be the same but they must also be consistent with the study's viewpoint. Rarely do CMA studies adopt a wide viewpoint but, as in all economic evaluations, the viewpoint must be explicit and easily understandable as it will dictate the study design and the type of inputs taken into consideration.

Types of costs included in CMA can vary from direct (those falling on the health care system for the production of the health intervention for the care of the condition considered) to indirect and intangible, as we have seen in the preceding chapter. As in all cases, all inputs must be identified, measured in natural units, and valued; the resulting methodological problems are common to all other study designs. A typical problem which occurs in CMA studies concerns the valuation of costs accruing in the future; this aspect, called time preference, is part of the current debate over discounting, which will be dealt with in some detail in Chapter 7. This debate, however, is concerned mainly with time adjustment of consequences.

A problem which we will examine in this example is that of apportioning *overhead costs*, defined as those, such as administration or heating and lighting, that are not linked directly to individual patient care but are nevertheless necessary to provide the intervention. There is no preferred method to apportion overheads, but the most common way in the past has been to divide the total running costs of, for example, a hospital, by the number of bed-days, thus calculating the cost per average patient per day. This is not really satisfactory as only "average" patients fit into this resource consumption model and investment costs of buildings and equipment may have been excluded from this equation. Readers should think through the decision to include or exclude such capital costs depending on the time frame for the decision. This is because, although such costs are fixed in the short run, they can vary in the long run.

Methods of cost apportionment are usually based on notional accountancy approaches, using reasonable knowledge about how particular resources such as heating, energy, or hospital portering services are provided and consumed. For example, heating is apportioned on the basis of a department's floor area or operating theatre use on the basis of time used, and so on. Obviously these methods, of which there are different types, require a considerable information system back-up and are quite complicated. The choice of method to allocate overheads must be made on the basis of the relative importance of the overheads to the total costs of the programme we are evaluating. As a general rule, when overheads are a small proportion of general costs, we can simplify apportioning by allocating to the intervention those costs which are unambiguously generated by the programme, discarding all costs of those resources which are not directly used by the intervention and apportioning what is left on the basis of volume of activity. A further principle would be to consider whether particular types of overhead cost would be completely unaffected by the alternative forms of care compared. In this case, it can be correct to exclude them from the analysis.

Scenario for cost-minimisation analysis

A busy DGH with numerous hypertensive patients in its catchment area who imposes a high resource burden for routine BP measurement. Initially there is a requirement to evaluate, through a randomised controlled trial design, whether home measurement of BP is as effective as GP measurement and, if so, which alternative is the cheapest. Analysis of the trial results shows that there is no difference in the effectiveness of the two procedures.

The monitoring of blood pressure and management of hypertension is a time-consuming activity for the hospital doctors and GPs working in St Crispin's and its catchment area. St Crispin's is a large DGH with a numerous population of people with hypertension who require frequent monitoring. Historically, attempts at reducing direct medical involvement for hypertension control have not been very successful. Home monitoring of BP (patient-administered) is an activity that many patients carry out as a complement to nurse BP reading but has never been conceived as a proper alternative and has never been evaluated as such.

Dr Baker, a consultant physician with many clinical trials under his belt, has received funding for a series of wide-ranging initiatives aimed at achieving better quality care for hypertensives. As part of this programme, Dr Baker aims to evaluate whether home BP assessment is a viable alternative to professional BP management. Additionally, he intends to calculate whether this system of BP monitoring is a cheaper alternative. He wants first of all to define whether the two alternatives produce the same consequences or not. As he is collecting data to get answers to these questions, he intends using the data to conduct an economic evaluation alongside his evaluation of consequences. If such consequences are the same, his economic evaluation will be a CMA design.

The GPs in his catchment area, whom he has involved in early discussions, are as eager to find an answer to the question, as BP monitoring workload rests mainly on their shoulders and that of their staff. They agree to recruit all their hypertensive patients into Baker's study and he excludes all those with cardiovascular complications who would make a different (higher) use of facilities at St Crispin's and in the community. Of the 94 GPs in his catchment area, 67 (71%) agree to take part in the study. Baker recruits 467 non-complicated hypertensive patients of which 430 accept to take part in the study. These he randomly assigns to a "home BP measurement" arm and to a "usual measurement" arm regardless of degree of hypertension and type of treatment.

Baker issues a small electronic BP measurement device to those subjects in the "home BP measurement" arm and carries out instruction sessions to enable the patients to use the device.

The patients in the "home BP measurement" arm are told to measure their BP twice weekly and record the readings on a chart, and every 4 weeks they must complete the chart, annotating variations in treatment and possible side-effects. The chart is then sent to the GP who also records the same data for their "usual measurement" arm patients. Dr Baker asks all GPs in the study to record the number of visits made by patients and the number of phone calls and chart mailings received. Dr Baker's research assistant is given the task of keeping track of outpatient consultations and the diagnostic procedures required. A copy of all the data is collected by Dr Baker's research assistant for the final BP measurement and evaluation.

At the beginning of the study all patients' BP is measured twice by the same expert nurse, Mrs Rose, and this is repeated at the end of the study a year later. For those subjects in the "home BP measurement" arm, Mrs Rose tests the concordance between the electronic device and her mercury sphygmomanometer. Every other month this procedure is repeated throughout the study on random samples of 20 patients.

Dr Baker aims to carry out statistical tests on the different tools of BP measurement throughout the study to exclude the possibility that final differences are due to the measurement tool.

Dr Baker had decided that the trial outcome measures will be the difference in BP from the baseline at the beginning of the trial for each arm, adjusted for age, gender and use of antihypertensives and the responses by patients and physicians to a satisfaction survey. He divides the resource items into those that may be common to both arms, such as primary care consultations, phone calls to the surgeries, and number of outpatient department visits (including diagnostic procedures) and those that are incurred only by the "home measurement" arm, such as the costs of the device, training, and mail.

Dr Baker realises that no hospital admissions linked to the study had taken place. To circumscribe the effect of the two monitoring regimes on resource use, Dr Baker decides to compare the use of resources in the year of the trial with the use made in the year preceding the trial which he had described with COI methodology in a sample survey. At the end of the trial Dr Baker's cohorts have fallen to 190 (88%) patients in the "usual measurement" arm and 200 (93%) in the "home BP measurement" arm.

Analysis of final trial data shows that there are no significant differences between patients in the two arms in terms of age, gender, race, education, initial BP, and percentage of patients on antihypertensive treatment.

BP control shows no significant difference between the two arms, with systolic BP having decreased by 1.4 mm Hg in the "home BP measurement" arm whereas it had risen by 1.8 mm Hg in the "usual measurement" arm. Diastolic readings showed respectively no change in the first group and an increase of 1.7 mm Hg in the second arm. These differences, which remained after adjusting for age, gender, race, baseline treatment, and BP, failed to reach statistical significance.

Patient and physician satisfaction was equally high in the two arms. GP time was called upon less by patients in the "home BP measurement" arm, and 86% of GPs thought that compliance with their advice was also higher in this arm.

The variation in resource use before and after the trial and between the two arms is shown in Table 4.1.

Table 4.1 Use of resources before, after and within the trial (average per patient)

Resource type BP	Prior to trial	Home BP	Trial usual
GP consultations	3.5	1.5	2.7
Telephone calls	0.7	1.5	0.8
Outpatient visits	0.8	0.9	0.7

When Dr Baker turns his attention to valuing resources used, he finds himself in a quandary. Firstly, he is unable to cost some items, in particular the cost of a visit to the outpatients department; secondly, he realises that his trial has involved possible disruption to the families of home BP measurements patients. This, he realises, may lead to extra costs which he has not accounted for. Additionally, one of his colleagues points out that the acquisition costs of the home measurement device cannot be used in its entirety, as the life of any such device is longer than the period of the trial.

In desperation, Dr Baker calls in Dr Stones, our well-known economist. Stones scolds Dr Baker, reminding him that the best time to involve an economist, or any other specialist, is at the study design stage when scientific questions can be framed appropriately and data collection can be tailored to answer the study question.

Stones, however, reassures Baker that all is not lost. Indirect costs, those accruing to the family, are likely to occur mostly to the "usual measurement" arm as these patients have a higher number of trips to the GP, leading to a greater expenditure in time and transport. If the CMA results already show the "home measurement" as the most convenient alternative, inclusion of indirect costs would only make it more so. Dr Baker's data however show no cases of time off work.

Next, Stones explains to Dr Baker how to cost all items. For phone calls and postal expenses he can use commercial tariffs. To cost GP and nurse time, Baker can use any one of a large number of published studies. Stones points out the best of a recent crop.

Baker's intention had been to cost outpatient attendances by taking the yearly running cost of the whole outpatient department and dividing it by the number of patients seen in a year.

Dr Stones is not happy with this approach as hypertensive patients are likely to use the facilities less intensively than other patients, and the use of what effectively is a capitation rate would lead to an overestimation of their outpatient costs. However, outpatient resource used by patients in each arm of the trial is not vastly different and there is little point in spending a lot of time in minutely defining the costs. Dr Stones proposes to identify in the outpatient database all resources, the use of which are directly attributable to hypertensive patients and to cost these resources, which are mainly diagnostic procedures, using estimates of shadow prices based on price information from private providers, but adjusted if there is evidence that the market price is not competitive.

Equally, Stones proposes the exclusion from the cost calculation of all items not directly used in the outpatient treatment of hypertensives, thereby excluding all capital investment costs and all costs relating to staff that do not come into contact with hypertensives. What is left of outpatient running costs is divided by the number of hypertensives seen.

Finally, Stones points out that acquisition and training costs for the measurement devices represent capital costs for the "home measurement" arm and he suggests the use of an annual discounted cost based on a 5-year useful life cycle of the device (see the footnote at the end of the chapter). As Baker's head is swimming by now, Stones suggests including a fifth of the costs in the equation, whereas as training was carried out by specially hired personnel, these are considered in full.

Having gathered the required data, Dr Baker calculates annual costs per patient in pounds sterling (1995) as shown Table 4.2.

Table 4.2   Dr Baker's calculations of costs per patient in pounds sterling (1995)

Resource	Trial arm	
	Home BP	Usual BP
GP consultations	34.8	64.9
Telephone calls	10.8	5.3
Outpatient visits	10.9	10.0
Total cost of hypertension management	56.5	80.2
Monitoring device	6.4	—
Training	1.3	—
Mail	3.6	—
Total cost of home monitoring	11.3	—
Total cost	67.8	80.2

Dr Baker now has a clear indication that home monitoring of BP is a more convenient alternative of a quality at least equal to the usual physician-based approach.

Dr Stones suggests finishing the study with what he calls a sensitivity analysis to test the robustness of the conclusions to the variation of some of the costs, especially the ones that have approximated. Dr Baker promises he will do this in his next study as he now has to marshal his arguments to convince all GPs and their hypertensive patients to switch to home monitoring and he is well aware that his economic argument is but one of the many points he will have to make to secure agreement.

Areas of controversy

Cost-minimisation is conceptually simple, as it compares the costs of alternative ways of achieving the same outcome, and as a consequence has not been subject to the controversies surrounding other forms of economic evaluation. However, the definition of a CMA is itself controversial, and it has been suggested that it should be considered a special case of CEA in which there is no evidence of difference in outcomes.

Another controversial issue relates to the level of research effort needed to estimate costs and whether a detailed cost analysis (as opposite to a less detailed one) leads to any practical difference in the conclusions of economic evaluations. This issue is relevant to all forms of economic evaluation—but particularly to CMA, where cost differences are the only reason for the decision about the best form of care. Very different standards are applied to the judgement of effectiveness evidence in health care evaluation (Guyatt *et al* 1995) than are applied to evidence of cost differences (Knapp and Beecham 1993) and, although sensitivity analysis is a valuable tool, work is still underway on methods to assess the level of confidence that can be attached to estimates of cost difference (Mugford 1996; Johnston *et al* 1999).

Footnote

Stones had recently estimated capital costs of equipment for a study of costs of electronic fetal monitoring in the labour ward. He showed this to Baker. He had used a method described by Drummond, O'Brien, Stoddart and Torrance (1997). He estimated an annual equivalent cost based on the current value, the expected life of 5 years, which determines the annual depreciation of value, 5% discount rate for future costs. The discount rate allows for the opportunity cost of lost interest from not investing the capital. He also included annual maintenance costs of one fifth of the initial capital value. Three levels of purchase cost were considered, to reflect the range of different models available (Table 4.3).

Table 4.3 Equipment for electronic fetal monitoring during labour (£ sterling)

Electronic monitor	Estimate	Low	High
Current value	8 000	5 000	10 000
Annual equivalent cost[a]	2 125	1 328	2 656
Annual maintenance	1 600	1 000	2 000
Total annual cost	3 725	2 328	4 656

[a]Taking account of depreciation and opportunity cost of capital, assuming a 5-year productive life and 5% discount rate (see Drummond *et al* 1997: (88–91).[2]

The estimated average annual cost per fetal monitor was just under half of the initial cost of the equipment. The average cost per woman monitored depends on the number of women who received electronic monitoring. The *marginal* cost of equipment for monitoring low-risk women was considered to be zero where equipment was already kept in the labour ward for use for the less frequent cases of high-risk labour, but became a net cost when a routine policy of electronic monitoring for all labour would require purchase of new machines.

Suggested reading

Drummond M, O'Brien B, Stoddart G, Torrance G. *Methods for the economic evaluation of health care programmes* (2nd edn.) Oxford: OUP, 1997.

Guyatt GH, Sackett DL, Sinclair JC, *et al*. Users' guides to the medical literature: a method for grading health care recommendations. *JAMA* 1995;**274**:1800–4. (A description of an approach to assessing the quality of evidence on effectiveness of interventions. This is helpful in deciding whether outcomes are really the same.)

Johnston K, Buxton M, Jones DR, Fitzpatrick R. Assessing the costs of health care technologies in clinical trials. *Health Technol Assess* 1999;**3**(6). (A review of the evidence about costing methods in health economics evaluation.)

Knapp M, Beecham J. Reduced list costings: examination of an informed short cut in mental health research. *Health Econ* 1993;**2**:312–22. (Costing methods can be quite simple and produce reliable results when compared to detailed methods—an example from community mental health.)

Soghikian K, Casper SM, Fireman BH, *et al*. Home blood pressure monitoring. Effects on use of medical services and medical care costs. *Med Care* 1992:**30**:855–65. (An example of a cost minimization study, the basis for the example used in this chapter.)

Research steps for a cost-minimisation analysis

Stage of economic evaluation	Example
Specification of the question, and baseline comparison group	To compare home blood pressure monitoring by patients with GP monitoring
Specification of the viewpoint, type and coverage of economic study	Evaluation from perspective of health providers and patients, effectiveness no different between options, therefore cost-minimisation analysis
Specification of key outcome and estimation of effectiveness	No key outcome because trial data showed no evidence of difference
Specification of method for valuation of health outcomes	Not relevant
Definition of costs to be estimated	GP visits, telephone calls, monitoring equipment, outpatient visits. Patient's time and travel not estimated because of evidence that this would not alter conclusion
Estimation of differences in quantities of resource use	Differences in use of services from randomised trial
Estimation of unit costs of elements of resource use	Commercial rates for phone calls, review of published evidence for health service costs for GPs. Opportunity costs of outpatient care estimated from adjusted private costs. Capital costs based on 5-year life, using annuitisation
Specification of analytic model	Simple comparison of average costs in two groups
Taking account of time preference	Short-term follow-up, no long-term costs to discount
Summarise economic result	Difference between average costs of alternatives
Sensitivity analysis	Not done at this stage, but highlighted as necessary

5 Cost-effectiveness analysis (CEA)

At times, alternative forms of care for a particular health problem may differ in the size of their effect on one or more health outcomes. However, if the principal effect on health can be satisfactorily expressed in a single dimension, such as mortality, then the alternative approaches to achieving a change in this outcome can be compared using cost-effectiveness analysis (or CEA for short). CEA is used to compare interventions which are broadly similar and adopts a narrower viewpoint (or perspective) than either CUA (see Chapter 6) or CBA (see Chapter 7).

The typical logical setting for CEA is that in which a decision to intervene on a particular problem has already been taken and CEA is carried out only in order to identify the most efficient way of achieving objective X. As we have seen in Chapter 1, it is for this reason that economists say that CEA is used to assess *technical* or *"X" efficiency*.

CEA, born in the 1960s, has quickly supplanted CBA in popularity up to the point where the term "cost-effectiveness analysis" is often used as synonymous with economic evaluation. This is a misleading use of economic terminology which causes confusion, especially in those who are not conversant with the full range of economic evaluation methodology. CEA should be regarded as a specific type of study design used to answer questions such as "what is the most efficient input to achieve a natural unit of outcome?" For example, to prevent one case of hepatitis A at least cost should we intervene with health education, good sanitation, γ-globulin, or vaccine? This would be answered in a CEA by comparing costs of these different interventions per avoided case (or per avoided death).

It is unusual for CEA to include indirect costs such as effects on productivity in the "wider economy". However, it is important that costs be considered beyond those of the sometimes narrow viewpoint and responsibility of the short-term health care provider. Costs can arise for patients and other agencies, both in the short and longer term. It is difficult to identify the point at which health care costs attributable to the form of health care in question or "direct costs", are divided from those that would arise anyway, but which differ as a result of life and are therefore indirect costs in addition to those indirect costs arising in the wider economy.

At times CEA includes costs both to health care providers and users which are used in cases when it is necessary to evaluate a wider impact of the intervention being assessed. For example, any mass screening campaign involves costs accruing to the families of the person or persons being screened (for example, time lost by mothers who take their children to the optician). Additionally, false test results generate anxiety and sometimes even expenses in an effort to reassure the screened person.

These changes in health care or other agencies' costs should be considered as arising from the programme of care. Anxiety and distress are also different dimensions of outcome, sometimes referred to as *intangible* (see also Chapter 3). These would be considered, if not actually measured in a CBA, and would ideally be reflected in utilities attached to each option in a CUA (see Chapter 6). If there are clear differences between two forms of care in such outcomes which are not the primary outcome in the evaluation, it would be good practice in CEA to report and comment on the evidence in the commentary.

Accounting for these costs as "side effects" and social costs is necessary, for example, when comparing different screening methods with different attendance requirements or false-positive rates. Their inclusion is a methodological shift as CEA still addresses only technical efficiency.

In CEA the relationship between inputs and consequences is expressed in terms of costs per natural unit such as case(s) avoided, hospital admissions avoided, dismissal from work or sickness absence avoided, life years gained, deaths avoided or cases identified (as in the case of a screening procedure). Obviously the expression of difference in impact on health in a CEA comparison between two forms of care is limited by the choice of the key health indicator used in the analysis. Where there is a clear trade-off between different

41

important outcomes (such as in the case of fewer deaths but increased numbers of disabled survivors after neonatal intensive care for very preterm babies) CUA or CBA should be preferred.

Because of the nature of questions typically addressed, CEA is the economic study design which is found most frequently alongside or nested within a randomised controlled trial (RCT). The two methodologies greatly benefit by their concurrent execution. The conclusions of RCTs are enhanced by the addition of a second perspective, that of economics. CEA, in turn, benefits from the least biased estimates of effectiveness deriving from RCTs and by the fact that resource data collected in RCTs are both individual and prospective, and therefore likely to be of higher quality than post hoc collections allow. A population perspective, or sample of it, also entails the calculation of actual costs and of their variability; this greatly enhances the possibility of generalising from them. It is therefore common for a CEA to be based on a synthesis of data from several sources, making assumptions as necessary about the compatibility of the data and testing these assumptions by varying them in sensitivity analysis (see below). A common format for such modelling is to use a decision analysis format, illustrating the choices and pathways of health care in a decision tree. Readers will find a brief introduction to decision analysis theory in Appendix 3 and a real life example of CEA based on available evidence in Chapter 8.

All calculations of inputs and consequences used in economic evaluations are based on uncertain size of effects, as our knowledge of the natural history of diseases and the effects of our interventions is imperfect. Additionally, uncertainty also relates to controversy in methods of economic evaluation (see discounting) and the possibility of transferring results from one economic evaluation in a specific setting to another setting.

At times the bracket of uncertainty surrounding the estimates in use in economic evaluation is such that conclusions may be overturned by the use of one extreme estimate instead of another. Because of this uncertainty it is common practice to examine the robustness of a result over a range of alternative estimates for uncertain parameters. These are usually varied one by one over a range of possible values. If the basic conclusions of the evaluation are not altered by changing a particular parameter, our confidence in the conclusions is increased. This formal procedure is called *sensitivity analysis*.

According to the number of parameters which are simultaneously varied, sensitivity analysis is defined as "one-way" or "two-way".

Different methods of varying these parameters further subdivide sensitivity analysis into:

- probabilistic, when the statistical distribution of the parameter is known and probabilities are used to calculate the likelihood of its occurrence;
- extreme, when the statistical distribution is unknown or estimates are calculated and in which only a few extreme values are used;
- threshold, when the decision cut-off point is known or needs to be defined and inputs and consequences are modelled accordingly to establish at what magnitude of the different cost or outcome variables the decision to adopt or reject the new form of care would be reversed.

There are few rules in applying sensitivity analysis, and there is no right answer as to which parameters should be varied, and how. As a consequence, sensitivity analysis is often criticised as being arbitrary and potentially biased. However, there is general agreement that it should be carried out and in an explicit manner.

Scenario for cost-effectiveness analysis

A maternity hospital with over 5000 annual births and a caesarean section rate of about 15% of deliveries which has a postoperative rate of wound infection of about 8% of all caesarean operations. Apart from the acute discomfort, women who experience wound infection have longer postnatal hospital stays, and require more intensive nursing care, together with antibiotic therapy and more laboratory tests than would normally be the case after a caesarean section. Robust evidence from systematic review of randomised trials suggests that the incidence of wound infection can be significantly reduced by a very short prophylactic course of antibiotics at the time of the operation. Adopting a policy of prophylactic antibiotics would reduce wound infection, but it is not clear at what additional cost, and whether, and under what conditions, this cost would be acceptable.

Miss Macgregor is a specialist in obstetrics who works in a large and very busy department with over 5000 deliveries a year at St Hilda's, an urban hospital. Miss Macgregor, influenced by one of her colleagues who is a member of the Cochrane Collaborative Review Group on Pregnancy and Childbirth, has been consulting the Cochrane Database of Systematic Reviews (CDSR) as she is trying to base her practice on up-to-date knowledge of the effectiveness of interventions. Specifically she has interrogated CDSR on the effectiveness of antibiotic prophylaxis immediately prior to or after caesarean section with the aim of decreasing the risk of wound infection. Miss Macgregor is aware that the onset of infection in a caesarean section wound usually means that the unfortunate mother and baby have a longer stay in hospital and sometimes experience serious complications, such as septicaemia. She is aware that her post-caesarean section wound infection rate is about 8.8%, which is above the estimated national average of 6%. Recently she has had two severe cases which necessitated hospital stays of several weeks in an isolation ward and the administration of intravenous antibiotics. These events have led Miss Macgregor to believe that, as pressure on obstetric beds is very high because of the closure of several nearby hospitals, any reduction of length of stay would increase bed availability.

Perusal of the CDSR reveals a systematic review of 69 controlled trials (comprising a population of 9207 women) in which patients' post-caesarean wound infection rates were compared after administration of a single dose or short course of antibiotics with placebo or no treatment. Although the original trials had slightly different end points, the review clearly demonstrated that the odds of wound infection were diminished by between 56% and 72% by routine administration of either of the two antibiotics, regardless of whether the operation had been carried out as an elective or an emergency one. This reduction in the odds of wound infection would imply a reduction from 8.8% to 4.4% in the wound infection rate after caesarean sections at St Hilda's. Differences between antibiotics appeared minimal from the analyses in the review.

Armed with this evidence, Miss Macgregor approaches Mr Slopers, the head of the obstetric unit, asking him to agree to the modification of treatment protocols to include the routine use of either broad-spectrum penicillins or cephalosporins to mothers undergoing delivery by caesarean section. Mr Slopers is less than enthusiastic about agreeing to Miss Macgregor's request as he cannot really understand this "evidence-based fad" (as he calls it). He is also honestly worried about the cost of such a practice and feels that he needs further evidence of the policy's desirability before he will agree to a change in protocol. This view is reinforced by the head of the finance department at St Hilda's.

Miss Macgregor, hiding her irritation at what she sees as a refusal to face facts, promises she will think about the problem. A few days later she coolly considers the main reasons for introducing routine antibiotic prophylaxis to be:

- to better the patient's lot;
- to release scarce resources (such as beds and staff time) for alternative use.

She quickly realises that the explicit introduction of an economic perspective may achieve the aim of convincing Mr Slopers of the justness of her cause (or at least deal with his objections).

She decides to ask the advice of Dr Stones, St Hilda's economist, who is known to her. Dr Stones swiftly sums up the problem and says to her: "You know, you are very lucky. You have a clear study question and a clear estimate of effect based on a large population of trials which have been rigorously reviewed, I wish I could say that of all researchers who come to me for help". Dr Stones advises Miss Macgregor that it would probably be sufficient initially to assess whether both or either antibiotic saved resources and, if so, by how much. An answer to the question of whether the drugs would increase the quality of life of patients or not should next be considered. If there is any evidence that one of the antibiotics affects quality of life differently from the other, the answer may be given by carrying out a CUA (see Chapter 6). In this case the systematic review indicates that there is no evidence of differential effect on quality of life, and a CUA, which is quite complicated, would probably be an overkill. In fact, if the prophylactic antibiotics work (as the review indicates), the quality of life of postoperative patients would certainly be enhanced by the absence of a wound infection. However, as the trials did not evaluate woman's views or breast-feeding problems, not all potential variables in the equation have been assessed, and Miss Macgregor and Dr Stones note this fact.

Stones advises Miss Macgregor that she should consider carrying out an economic evaluation using the framework of CEA to:

- assess whether and in what circumstances additional costs are associated with the gain in outcome from antibiotic prophylaxis;
- assess whether resources are saved by the routine use of antibiotic prophylaxis in elective and emergency caesarean sections, and
- test the sensitivity of the results to the use of cephalosporins instead of ampicillin as the antibiotic used for prophylaxis.

Dr Stones frames the two questions as a logical sequence. Firstly does the routine use of antibiotics save resources or not? If the answer is no, this may be due to the fact that only direct cost have been taken into account. It is then likely that Miss Macgregor may have to attempt a more complicated form of economic evaluation with the introduction of quality-of-life measures, indirect costs (such as productivity losses) or intangible costs (such as disruption to family life by the increased stay of mother and child in hospital). These would need to be considered before deciding not to use antibiotics routinely.

However, if the answer to the second question is yes, quality-of-life measures and intangible costs would need to be taken into consideration only if it is expected that side effects might outweigh the benefits of reduced infection, as the antibiotics are worth introducing routinely anyway. At this point, however, it is necessary to assess which antibiotic is the cheapest to use in order to decrease the risk of a post-caesarean wound infection.

Miss Macgregor, struck by the logic of such a chain of thought, decides to attempt gathering data to answer the first study question. St Hilda's has a good ICD-based patient information system, and Miss Macgregor soon learns that, in the preceding 6 months, 486 patients were delivered by caesarean section. Miss Macgregor checked a sample of case notes and found that in cases where infection was mentioned in the notes, a full course of antibiotics had been prescribed and that no patients were given prophylactic antibiotics.

Next comes the problem of how to define a wound infection. The only practicable way forward appears to be to accept "mention of a wound infection in the notes" (and hence on the coded database) as proof of infection. Miss Macgregor feels that this solution is rather broad and is less rigorous than some of the end-points of the trials in the review which, for instance, had to have laboratory confirmation of the infection as a definition of outcome of the trial. Dr Stones advises her that use of such a broad definition additionally carries the risk of overestimating the incidence of infection at St Hilda's and hence overestimating the potential consequences of routine use of antibiotics. Both researchers, however, agree that as long as the problems associated with choosing such a definition are made explicit in the study report, the course of action they have chosen is reasonable. Additionally, as they near the conclusion of the study, their intention is to test the robustness of their findings by assuming different effectiveness levels and staff costs and carrying out a sensitivity analysis.

Miss Macgregor and Dr Stones turn their attention to what is known from the information system about patients who undergo caesarean section and those who subsequently have a wound infection. They sum up their findings by listing *the mean* length of stay (in days) at St Hilda's of women who undergo caesarean section:

Uncomplicated section	6.7
Section with wound infection	8.8
Difference	2.1

As the probability of the difference between the means having occurred by chance is less than 0.004 (very small), the difference is very likely to be real

Next, they itemise and calculate the resources and unit costs for all patients who have undergone caesarean section, further subdividing them into patients with and without wound infection, thus working out the differential costs of infection. To do this they turn to the midwifery notes and records of a random sample of 200 of the 486 patients augmented by the observation or practice in the ward. To determine unit costs they use figures available from the finance department of St Hilda's and from its pharmacy and laboratory. Their calculations are summarised in Tables 5.1 and 5.2 which show costs per patient rounded to the nearest unit.

Macgregor and Stones now calculate the costs of the interventions. These are taken as equal to the acquisition costs of a course of proprietary ampicillin and cefoxitin (£4.10 and £49 respectively).

Next, the two researchers model the incremental costs, per case avoided, of routine use of antibiotics on a hypothetical cohort of 100 patients. They do this by assuming an 8.4% infection rate and using the formula:

Cost = (cost per patient without infection × number of patients without infection) + (cost of patient with infection × number of patients with infection)

Table 5.1 Cost per patient with infection at St Hilda's, broken down by resource quantity and type and unit cost

	Patients with infection			
	Resources			
	Type	Quantity	Unit cost (£)	Total cost (£)
Staffing				
Medical	Hours	3.2	38	123
Midwifery	Hours	46.7	17	795
Microbiology	Test	3.5	3.7	13
Materials	Sundry[a]	19.5	2.3	45
Hotel costs	Days	8.8	45	400
Other	Sundry[b]	—	—	60
Total				1436

[a] These are averaged across sundry materials.
[b] For brevity, several items such as administration, physiotherapy, and so on are grouped within this item.

Table 5.2   Cost per patient with and without infection at St Hilda's and differential costs

	Patients with infection (£)	Patients without infection (£)	Increased cost due to infection (£)
Staffing			
Medical	123	91	32
Midwifery	795	250	545
Microbiology	13	6	7
Materials	45	24	21
Hotel costs	400	304	96
Other	60	45	15
Total	1436	720	716

At this point they devise a simple decision tree to represent their model (see Figure 5.1).

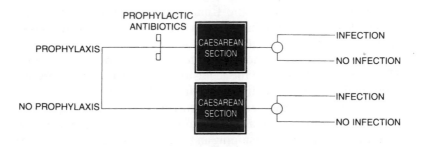

Figure 5.1   *Decision model for antibiotic prophylaxis at caesarean section.*

Assuming a mean 60% effectiveness of prophylactic antibiotics and all patients to be covered by prophylaxis, then there will be 5 (3.4 fewer) infected patients in the cohort. The cost per unit of incremental saving for each treatment cohort will be as shown in Table 5.3.

Table 5.3   Cost per unit of incremental saving for each antibiotic treatment cohort in Mr Sloper's department

	Input (Drug costs)	Effects (Change in health care savings)	Ratio (Cost per unit of incremental saving)
Ampicillin	£ 41	–£2434	0.017
Cefoxitin	£490	–£2434	0.201

As the effectiveness of both antibiotics assessed by the review varied between 50% and 70%, they recalculate their results according to the two extreme levels of prophylactic antibiotic policy. This procedure is known as a *one-way sensitivity analysis*. The analysis shows that routine prophylaxis, even when we adopt the most expensive antibiotic with a 50% assumption, is cost-saving. The most beneficial results are obtained by routine use of ampicillin at 70% effectiveness (Table 5.4).

Table 5.4   One-way sensitivity analysis varying antibiotic effectiveness estimates

	Reduction in odds of infection (%)	Estimated change in costs (£/100 caesarean sections)
Ampicillin	50	–2,707
	70	–3,938
Cefoxitin	50	–1,300
	70	–2,532

As the main cost driver is the difference in midwifery personnel time, and considering the potential variability of this cost between settings of care, Stones suggests introducing a *two-way sensitivity analysis* to test the robustness of their results to variation in effectiveness *and* midwifery staff time (Table 5.5).

Table 5.5   Two-way sensitivity analysis varying antibiotic effectiveness estimates and midwifery staff time

	Reduction in rate of infection (%)	Total cost (£/100 sections)	Estimated change (£/100 sections)
	(assuming daily additional cost of midwifery of £53)		
None	—	77 878	
Ampicillin	50	75 171	–2,707
	70	73 940	–3,938
Cefoxitin	50	76 578	–1,300
	70	75 346	–2,532
	Reduction in rate of infection (%)	Total cost (£/100 sections)	Estimated change (£/100 sections)
	(assuming daily additional cost of midwifery of £7.85)		
None	—	74 541	
Ampicillin	50	73 502	–1,039
	70	72 946	–1,595
Cefoxitin	50	74 909	+368
	70	74 353	–188

These tables show total costs which include the costs of the antibiotics for the cohort.

In only one scenario of these sensitivity calculations does the policy of antibiotic prophylaxis increase costs. This is the case of using cefoxitin at lower assumed effectiveness with the lower estimated difference in midwifery cost. Head-to-head trials have shown that cephalosporins, of which cefoxitin is one example, do not have any advantage over broad-spectrum penicillins as prophylaxis at caesarean section. Therefore, unless necessary for other reasons, the additional cost is not justified. If it were justified, the cost-effectiveness ratio, or additional cost per additional case of wound infection prevented, would be £70. It is not necessary to estimate the cost-effectiveness ratio where health outcomes are improved and costs reduced. In this case overall efficiency is necessarily improved by adopting the new form of care: it is said to be a dominant form of care.

In conclusion, at the highest level of sensitivity, that of answering the question of whether antibiotics are worth introducing routinely, the answer is unequivocally yes. In other words, regardless of which antibiotic is used, its estimated effectiveness, and the costs likely to be avoided, routine use of antibiotics is cost-saving (except when cefoxitin is used at 50% effectiveness with low midwifery costs). However, the results are said to be sensitive to the choice of antibiotic, as ampicillin appears to be the best buy throughout.

Miss Macgregor and Dr Stones have not quite finished their study yet as they should take into consideration other costs of the routine use of antibiotics such as possible onset of resistance and possible side effects from their use. They estimate that at an infection rate of 8.0%, a single-dose policy for prophylaxis (which is demonstrated to be as effective as the longer courses) would in fact reduce the number of cases requiring antibiotic treatment, and the total patient-days of antibiotics in women having post-caesarean care at St Hilda's would be less than without prophylaxis.

Side effects certainly impose real costs but are very difficult to measure and value. The most common manifestation is a rash which appears in approximately 5% of patients and which may lead to a change in antibiotic. Its effect on patients' utility would probably be determined only with a prospective survey based on preference measurement for different relevant health states. It would be possible to extend the decision model shown in Figure 5.1 to include a further subdivision of outcomes, adverse drug reaction or no adverse drug reaction, which would follow either infection or no infection after either form of care. The weights that patients attach to each of these states could be assessed using utility measurement methods (see Chapter 6).

Another problem is that of the external validity of such a study. How representative is St Hilda's, and how do marginal costs in this setting compare to those of other obstetric departments? The use of an isolation ward, for instance, may or may not be standard practice in other hospitals. This is another difficult question to answer and appears to Miss Macgregor and Dr Stones to transcend the aim of the study. Our researchers decide to mention these issues in the text without any attempt at solving them.

Mr Slopers is still not completely convinced by the evidence that Miss Macgregor produces but he is willing to back a prospective cohort study on the incidence of post-caesarean wound infection. Miss Macgregor is now busy organising this. She has also been alerted to possible longer-term differences in costs and outcomes after discharge from hospital and will work with the community midwives to assess the incidence of infection occurring for the first time after hospital discharge and will consider whether there is any evidence of an increase in delayed infectious morbidity in women receiving prophylaxis. She has found that as she now has a powerful analytical framework, she can vary the quantity of inputs (the type of antibiotic for instance) and see what the effect on the net cost-effectiveness balance is. Miss Macgregor, in other words, is planning to use the framework of the sensitivity analysis to play "what if...".

Areas of controversy

One of the most important controversies in recent years has been centred on the role and design of CEA. Specifically, economists have argued about whether to calculate and include certain costs (such as indirect ones) in the CEA study design on the cost side.

Many economists consider that CEA is not an economic evaluation according to the theoretical model of welfare economics—which considers overall economic welfare gained from different allocations of society's resources.

In general, if one has decided that CEA is not a form of economic evaluation in tune with welfare economics, then the issue of whether it should or should not include certain costs or outcomes on theoretical grounds becomes less valid. However, if the costs or outcomes are omitted from a CEA, then it is also incorrect to draw fundamental conclusions about overall economic efficiency from the study.

Readers should make up their own mind on whether cost not directly falling to the health service should be included or not, but should make their choice explicit and present costs broken down by category.

Readers should also be aware that, at times, North American economists use the term CEA to include both CMA and CUA.

Suggested reading

Briggs AH, Gray AM. Handling uncertainty. In economic evolution of health care interventions. *BMJ* 1999, **319**:635–8. (A good methodological review of the topic).

Briggs AH, Sculpher A, Buxton M. Uncertainty in the economic evaluation of health-care technologies: the role of sensitivity analysis. *Health Econ* 1994;**3**:95–104. (Authoritative and clear position paper on the rationale for and the role of sensitivity analysis.)

Cochrane Collaboration. *The Cochrane database of systematic reviews*. In: Cochrane Collaboration. *Cochrane Library*. Oxford: Update Software (CD-ROM).

Ludbrook A. The cost-effectiveness of the treatment of chronic renal failure. *Appl Econ* 1981;**13**:340–50. (CEA, based on decision analysis taking account of changes in health state over time, in a simply described Markov model. This study is based on nationally relevant data, and provides a basis for updating, using more recent estimates of the costs and probabilities for different options and health states.)

Mugford M, Hutton G, Fox-Rushby J, on behalf of the Steering Group for the WHO Antenatal Care Trial. Methods for economic evaluation alongside a multi-centre trial in developing countries: a case study from the WHO antenatal care trial. *Paediat Perinat Epidemiol* 1998:**12** (Suppl 2):75–97. (This paper describes the methods to be used for a cost-effectiveness study alongside an international multicentre randomised trial.)

Mugford M, Kingston J, Chalmers I. Reducing the incidence of infection after caesarean section: implications of prophylaxis with antibiotics for hospital resources. *BMJ* 1989;**299**:1033–6. (The example in this chapter was based on this study.)

Smith TJ, Hillner BE. The efficacy and cost-effectiveness of adjuvant therapy of early breast cancer in pre-menopausal women. *J Clin Oncol* 1993;**11**:771–6. (Example of a cost-effectiveness analysis based on systematic review of clinical trials and decision modelling approach.)

Research steps for a cost-effectiveness analysis

Stage of economic evaluation	Example
Specification of the question, and baseline comparison group	Women who have caesarean section with antibiotic prophylaxis, compared with no routine prophylaxis
Specification of the viewpoint, type and coverage of economic study	Short-term, health providers perspective in one maternity hospital
Specification of key outcome and estimation of effectiveness	Post-caesarean infection, evidence of effectiveness from review of RCTs, applied to local incidence of infection in the absence of antibiotic prophylaxis
Specification of method for valuation of health outcomes	Not relevant in CEA
Definition of costs to be estimated	Costs of prophylactic antibiotics, hospital postnatal care costs
Estimation of differences in quantities of resource use	Doses of prophylaxis required, days of stay in hospital, additional treatment costs for care of cases of infection. Hospital clinical activity statistics for baseline data on infection rates and lengths of stay

continued

Estimation of unit costs of elements of resource use	Observation of inputs to care for women with wound infection, additional data from case notes, supplies, equipment and CSSD departments. Hospital accounting data for average hotel and overhead costs of postnatal care, pharmacy and laboratories for costs of antibiotics and tests. Difference in costs estimated as product of unit costs and difference in use of resources for each policy per 100 women
Specification of analytic model	Decision analysis
Taking account of time preference	Time period is less than a year, so discounting is not necessary
Summarise economic result	Comparison of changes in costs and wound infection rates. Compare cost differences, if costs are increased, consider estimating incremental cost of additional health gain
Sensitivity analysis	Multiple one-way sensitivity analysis for initial incidence of infection, costs of postnatal care, costs (and types) of antibiotic

6 Cost-utility analysis (CUA)

As we have seen, CEA is particularly useful when we need to choose among alternative forms of care for the same problem. CEA is, however, less useful when the consequences of different interventions are different, and especially when such interventions cause differences simultaneously in the quality of life and the quantity of survival. This type of consequence is not rare in health interventions.

To overcome this complex problem, the last two decades have seen an increase in interest in the development of utility-based measures of consequence.

"Utility" is a term used by economists to signify what a person expects to gain from the consumption of a good or service. This concept is applied in health care to mean the individual's preference for different states of well-being deriving from the use of health care interventions.

Although the most correct method of measuring utilities is the contingent valuation approach, this suffers from a number of practical problems (see Chapter 7). The most commonly used measures are therefore estimated by weighting the changes in different mutually exclusive health states by their relative utilities, as judged in surveys of representative groups of people. The most famous utility is the QALY—pronounced "qualy", which is based on a quantity of life scale adjusted for its quality.

The example in this chapter calculates consequences by assessing health levels and applying utility values derived from preferences of population samples, as in the Rosser and Watts matrix (see below). There are alternatives to this type of calculation which construct utilities in a direct manner, by eliciting patients' preferences face to face. There are three widely used approaches.

The first approach is the *rating scale measurement* where a subject is asked to place his/her current health status on a line that goes from 0 (death) to 1 (perfect health).

The second is the *time trade-off (TTO)* measurement in which the subjects, on the basis of their current health status, have to decide how many years of his remaining life expectancy they would like to exchange for complete health. This is traditionally thought to be simple to administer.

The last approach is the *standard gamble* measurement, based on utility theory, in which individuals have to choose between living the rest of life in their current state or a gamble (for instance a surgical procedure) which, if won, will mean perfect health and, if lost, will signify death. The probability of the gamble paying off is changed until there is indifference between the probability of the two events. This probability expresses the individual's preference for his or her health state.

As can be seen, these direct measures are not easily applied and used, and readers are advised to consult an economist prior to an attempt at using such methodology.

Whichever way they are derived, these preferences are used to construct weighted measures of consequence such as the QALY. QALYs are calculated simply by multiplying the value of preference of being in a certain state by the length of time of being in that state. In choosing the method to use to measure QALYs, two factors must be considered: how health status will be measured (will it be a generic health status questionnaire, or a disease specific measure?), and whose "preference weights" will be attached to these health states (will it be representative of the population or of the patients who are likely to experience the intervention?). The answer depends on the viewpoint of the evaluator. If the evaluation is intended to provide evidence about the incremental cost per QALY of the intervention, in order to compare it with other options for health spending, then a generic, representative measure is needed.

One instrument, which has been developed by a collaborative team of European researchers, is the EuroQol or EQ-5D. The EuroQol is one of several instruments which measure health status in different domains (in the case of EuroQol these are: mobility, self-care, usual activities, pain/discomfort, anxiety/depression), and then apply preferences derived (using the TTO method in the case of

EuroQol), from large population-based studies. This relatively simple approach is quite widely used and available to researchers, and is being validated in different contexts.

An alternative is the healthy year equivalent (HYE) which uses a two-stage lottery method and which may represent better individual preferences. The theoretical basis for this method has been debated (Johannesson *et al* 1993; Mehrez and Gafni 1993). Johannesson and colleagues suggest the HYE approach is the same as the time trade-off method for QALY estimation. It is early to say how much practical difference to the estimation of cost-utility is made by different methods.

QALYs assume that the subject's preference for a state of health is independent of the time spent in that state. This may not always be true as minor conditions are likely to be borne better as time goes on, whereas serious conditions are less likely to be. To construct HYEs, subjects are briefed on the whole natural history of the diseases, thus removing the problem. CUA is a specialised variant of CEA in which consequences are expressed in utilities (such as QALYs) instead of in natural units as in CEA. Utilities express individual preference as judgements of the relative value of the consequences of interventions. As such, a cost-utility evaluation is an attempt to compare the consequences of intervening on different illnesses and conditions. In this sense it is an attempt at aiding the decision-making process which leads to allocative decisions in health-care. This is the most controversial aspect of CUA, as many economists and doctors do not accept the comparability of utilities arising from different measurement instruments, health problems and interventions. These issues will be dealt with at the end of this chapter.

Scenario for cost-utility analysis

The intensive care unit of a large teaching hospital with a high pressure on the availability of beds and the possibility that patients admitted with serious health problems, such as haemorrhagic stroke, may be adequately treated in non-ICU beds. Such a treatment decision would release scarce ICU beds for patients who would benefit from a stay in the ICU. The problem is to design a study which would assess the difference in both quantity and quality of life in haemorrhagic stroke patients comparing both costs and outcomes of their stay in ICU and non-ICU beds.

A young anaesthetist called Dr Spooner, who works in the intensive care unit of a large teaching hospital, is convinced that his department has insufficient beds. Dr Spooner, however, also believes that this is due partly to wrong use of those available. On the basis of his experience, Spooner knows that seriously ill patients are difficult to re-assign to beds other than those in the ICU. However, some serious problems, such as haemorrhagic stroke, are dealt with in a wholly rational manner, and patients admitted with symptoms suggestive of such a problem are processed on the basis of bed availability, time of arrival, relatives' wishes, and so on. There is little in the literature on the classification of such patients and on the clinical effectiveness of intensive treatment. In these circumstances the possibility of inappropriate use of beds is very high. Stroke patients who could be adequately treated in other wards are admitted to the ICU without considering the opportunity costs of such actions, i.e. excluding one or more patients who would benefit more from ICU admission.

Spooner carries out a literature review, looking for studies which would help him to maximise the use of his ICU beds but only finds a few COI studies and a few incomplete evaluations which his economist friend Dr Stones tells him are methodologically poor. Dr Spooner decides to carry out his own study, looking for a design which would allow him to consider all the different consequences on the quantity and quality of life which are produced by ICU interventions. He settles for CUA. He decides to use one main diagnosis as a marker for the many with which his patients are admitted. He is aware that this will restrict the scope of his study but will allow him to look at inputs and consequences of alternative ways of dealing with haemorrhagic stroke.

Spooner's first step is to define an adequate comparator, and he defines this as the best alternative treatment to ICU admission when this is not available.

He next considers whether he should carry out a retrospective or prospective study design. Initially his intention is to carry out a prospective study which assigns patients randomly to the ICU or to the best alternative. However, his local clinical epidemiologist, Professor Florence, points out the ethical and logistical problems which such a design would entail. It is very difficult to deny a patient an available ICU bed on the basis of random allocation. In addition, prospective recruitment is time-consuming.

Dr Spooner opts for a retrospective design, even though he is aware that the comparability of groups is an important issue. For instance, he decides not to include in the study stroke admissions with signs of respiratory distress, which, on the basis of regional guidelines, must be admitted to the nearest ICU. He knows that stroke cases who are not admitted to the ICU are admitted to the general medical ward, so he decides that these cases will form the comparator. In the 1995 ICU database he identifies 27 patients who have been admitted with a diagnosis of haemorrhagic stroke (ICD 9 431–2); 15 of these died during admission while of the remainder, six are still alive at the 6-month follow-up according to their GP.

Through the medical ward records he traces 18 stroke cases, of which 10 died during admission and five were still alive at the 6-month follow-up (see Table 6.1).

Table 6.1   Outcomes for patients with haemorrhagic stroke by comparison groups

	Intensive care	Medical ward
Patients admitted	27	18
Died during admission	15	10
Alive at 6-month follow-up	6	5

Dr Spooner now examines the clinical details of his patients. He realises that, as there is considerable diversity in the gravity of the cases, probably the most correct approach would be to stratify patients according to the seriousness of their condition. Additionally he decides to apply the simplified acute physiology score, or SAPS, to assign each case to an appropriate severity stratum and facilitate comparison between the two groups.

He swiftly realises, however, that, with such a small group of patients, stratification implies very small numbers in each stratum, severely limiting the level of confidence which can be attached to Spooner's study. At the same time he discards the idea of using conjoint analysis, a sophisticated method which allows assessment of all characteristics (including non-healthcare related) of a service being provided. Its use had been suggested by Dr Stones to assess the preferences of patients and their relatives. As conjoint analysis can only assess a limited number of variables, Spooner and Stones, on further reflection, decided against using such a method. Dr Spooner is not disheartened as he will use the study as a pilot to learn CUA methodology and build upon it at a later date.

At this stage Dr Spooner has to choose the method he will use to measure consequences. He asks his epidemiologist which ideal qualities he should look for in a measure of consequences. The answer is that the method should be applicable to all patients, encompass all main aspects of quality of life and allow comparison of quality of life among different groups of patients to be made. It must also be reproducible among the same patients, sensitive enough to detect important changes in the clinical status of patients, use the same methods of calculation, and should be easy to use.

Dr Spooner realises that such an ideal measure does not exist and decides that he will use a traditional instrument which estimates length of life and adjusts it for quality. He decides to use mortality rates and survival (in years) as natural measures and to adjust them for quality of life at 6-month follow-up compared to quality of life before the stroke. He will build up a picture of pre-stroke quality of life by talking to patients and their families at the 6-month follow-up. This will entail the possibility of recall bias, but is the only feasible way of achieving the goal. He will approximate the pre-stroke quality of life of deceased patients, which is of course impossible to calculate directly, by assuming that it is equal to that of survivors.

He now talks to Professor Florence and finds out that there are other disease-specific and generic instruments of quality measurement. Disease-specific instruments assess those dimensions of quality of life which are most directly affected by the specific disease. Dr Spooner has, however, failed to find any specific measures for stroke. Generic measures cover the main dimensions of quality of life (physical function, self-care, pain, psychological status, and social integration) and can be applicable to all diseases and be used to compare healthy subjects with patient populations.

Dr Spooner decides to use one of the most famous and widely used scales, the disability/distress scale designed by Rosser and Watts in 1972 and derived from a population of 70 interviewees (Table 6.2). This assesses quality of life under two dimensions: disability (objective dysfunction and physiological limitation due to illness) and distress (individual psychological reaction to illness). Each patient is assessed according to four levels of distress and eight levels of disability. Each combination of levels of distress and disability is reflected in a health state to which a value is attached; the values range from below 0 for a state worse than death, to 0 (death) to 1 (perfect health).

Usually, quality of life status is judged on the basis of the distress and disability combination through the medium of an intermediate questionnaire, called health measurement physical questionnaire

Table 6.2   Disability/distress scale designed by Rosser and Watts in 1972

Disability	Distress			
	A (none)	B (mild)	C (moderate)	D (severe)
I (none)	1.000	0.995	0.990	0.967
II (slight social disability)	0.990	0.986	0.973	0.932
III (severe social disability)	0.980	0.972	0.956	0.912
IV (performance severely limited)	0.964	0.956	0.942	0.870
V (no paid employment or education)	0.946	0.935	0.900	0.700
VI (chair-bound)	0.875	0.845	0.680	0.000
VII (bedridden)	0.677	0.564	—	−1.486
VIII (unconscious)	−1.028	not applicable		

(HMPQ) which enables each subject through his or her answers to be assigned a value on the Rosser and Watts scale.

Dr Spooner stratifies his responses on the basis of three SAPS levels, calling them groups 1 (SAPS less than 10 for patients who are not seriously ill), 2 (SAPS between 10 and 15) and 3 (SAPS over 15, for seriously ill patients). Once he has consolidated his answers the matrix looks like that in Table 6.3.

By multiplying each patient's post-stroke reduced life expectancy by the appropriate quality of life values in the Rosser and Watts matrix, Dr Spooner derives a utility measure which he calls QALE (quality-

Table 6.3   Dr Spooner's three SAPS levels by group

Group	Indicators	Intensive care	Medical ward
Group 1	Patients	8	12
	% dead	62.5	62.0
	Pre/post stroke QOL difference	−0.048	−0.210
	Average SAPS value	8.37	6.16
Group 2	Patients	9	6
	% dead	77.7	100
	Pre/post stroke QOL difference	−0.022	nil
	Average SAPS value	14.10	12.5
Group 3	Patients	10	nil
	% dead	90.0	nil
	Pre/post stroke QOL difference	−0.010	nil
	Average SAPS value	19.10	nil

adjusted life-expectancy). The average reduction of QALE after the stroke for the three SAPS groups of patients is shown in Table 6.4.

Table 6.4   Average QALE reduction of life after stroke according to Dr Spooner's calculations

SAPS groups	Patients	Intensive care	Medical ward
Less than 10	Dead	−34.47	−17.66
	Survived	−1.26	−0.96
10 to 15	Dead	−22.56	−11.99
	Survived	−1.28	nil
Over 15	Dead	−32.59	nil
	Survived	−0.01	nil

Now Dr Spooner turns his attention to inputs and decides that he will take a societal viewpoint as this is consistent with his original aim which was to facilitate a rational use of ICU beds in a public institution. He should therefore also take into consideration indirect costs such as the ones falling on families. He decides from this perspective that, as the groups are broadly comparable, indirect costs falling on families are likely to be of similar magnitude and can be omitted. He will calculate only direct health care costs.

As Dr Spooner's hospital does not produce cost centre estimates of services used, he decides to use a set of assumptions to approximate costs. Through their medical records he identifies resources used by his patients as follows:

- those interventions which require only equipment which is in general use and personnel time;
- those interventions which require consumables;
- laboratory and radiodiagnostics;
- drugs.

The values of these resources he assigns as follows:

- for those interventions which require only equipment which is in general use and personnel time—nil, as the opportunity cost of these resources is negligible;
- for those interventions which require consumables he calculates only acquisition costs;
- for laboratory and radiodiagnostics he uses a private hospital price list. Dr Stones' suggestion of adopting this approach for this item leads Dr Spooner to use the "shadow price" of these items.

Dr Stones points out that as we have no idea of what the production costs of these items are within Spooner's hospital, he should look at the acquisition costs of these goods from an outside provider, such as the private sector. This assumes that production capacity within the hospital is at saturation point so that any extra activity has to be bought in. As this is not likely to be the case, shadow prices are likely to be an overestimate of the true costs. Dr Spooner calculates drug costs on the basis of their acquisition costs, but he also realises that he has failed to consider differential use of community services, such as rehabilitation in the first 6 months, and use of the medical ward by recovering ICU patients. He decides to add personnel, equipment, and general (power, water, heating, maintenance) costs. He derives the latter from total hospital budget costs and attributed by length of stay in days. For personnel he considers budget costs only for the two departments involved in the study (see Table 6.5).

Table 6.5   Dr Spooner's estimates of costs (in 1995 pounds sterling) for stroke patients

Costs per sector	Intensive care	Medical ward
Treatment	22 838	2 066
Personnel	78 454	7 670
Major equipment	6 066	140
Overheads	48 840	73 555
Total	156 198	83 431

There is a striking difference between costs in the two departments for all sectors, but particularly for personnel and treatment.

Dr Spooner would like to calculate the incremental costs per QALE for the ICU compared to the medical ward but this small and diverse sample of patients does not allow him to carry out a direct comparison. Dr Stones and Professor Florence are so struck by the results that they suggest addressing the problems of a small sample through the means of a model. This would allow exploration of the possible range of consequences given different levels of the problem and of costs and effectiveness.

Their idea is to apply Dr Spooner's unit costs to a simulated population of patients with the same SAPS level. However, even this model is not feasible as there are insufficient reliable data on the gravity and occurrence of stroke in the population. They decide to construct a model by standardising patient categories by severity of illness. They model three control groups for each SAPS level with the same clinical characteristics of ICU patients to whom they apply mortality and QOL measures of the medical ward patients. The calculation of incremental costs is now done directly in QALYs as patients have been standardised and have the same life expectancy.

The results of this simulation show that patients with SAPS lower than 10 (the least ill) benefit most from medical ward treatment and have the lowest cost per QALY (£3136). In the next group (SAPS 10 to 15) the results show the opposite, with maximum benefit in the ICU and a small differential cost (£190 per QALY). For the third group (SAPS more than 15) they assume that there is no alternative treatment, and the benefit from the ICU is 16.5 QALYs, with an incremental cost of £2778 per QALY.

The same simulation model is used to carry out a sensitivity analysis suggested by Dr Stones who is not absolutely happy with the quality of cost data used in the study.

Laboratory and diagnostic costs in particular, which are based on private sector prices, may not reflect the true marginal value of such

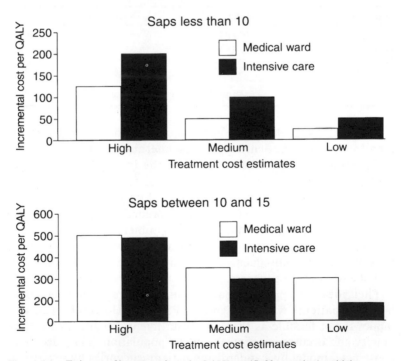

Figure 6.1   *Estimates of incremental cost for QALY stratified by severity (sensitivity analysis)*

procedures in their hospital. To test the robustness of the study's conclusions to the variation in such costs, Dr Stones suggests using a low cost estimate (calculated by halving the list price) and a high estimate (calculated by doubling the initial cost).

In Figure 6.1, Drs Spooner and Stones give a graphic representation of low, medium, and high estimates of incremental costs per QALY in patients with SAPS values below 10 and in those with SAPS values between 10 and 15. The most convenient intervention is still admission to the medical ward in less serious cases and intensive care in more serious cases, although the difference in incremental costs per QALY is sensitive to the cost estimates used.

Attending a world congress on intensive care 6 months later, Dr Spooner presents his conclusions: that all patients with SAPS indices above 10 should be directly admitted to the ICU, thereby maximising the use of scarce beds.

Conclusions

We have deliberately picked an example which demonstrated the original role of CUA, that of being a CEA capable of weighting consequence measures for quality of life. Our example is set in a scenario which makes this consideration of paramount importance.

Areas of controversy

Utilities exercise considerable appeal for decision-makers as they allow the quantification of different consequences of varied interventions undertaken on different problems. Utilities have been used in so-called QALY league tables in which different interventions are put into cost-per-QALY order in an effort to clarify "best buy" strategies. Such an allocative aim has attracted considerable interest and criticisms.

Perhaps the largest and most famous example of the use of CUA in an allocative role has been the Oregon experiment where the original programme had the aim of prioritising 1600 health problems on the basis of the cost-utility ratio deriving from interventions to deal with them. Preferences were measured on the basis of 30 different health states assessed in a telephonic survey of 1000 inhabitants. Because of a series of problems linked with data validity, the programme was restricted to a third of the original conditions and to three health states. Many other similar attempts have taken place, albeit of a more limited nature.

The debate on the role of cost-utility league tables is still raging, but the prevailing view is that they should be treated with extreme caution. Criticisms are based on the observation that the original studies (so-called "primary" studies) from which cost-utility estimates are derived are often methodologically weak. Primary studies have often been carried out in a different era, looking at different technologies and prices and with unreliable data. The capability of generalising across contexts, which QALY league tables are founded on, is limited by the differences in the frequency of illness, by the offer of health services, and by the type of health service organisation available. Other criticisms centre around the inequitable effect on the elderly and other categories that some league tables exercise. Equally, some health status measures have design weaknesses and some others cannot compare consequences credibly.

All such criticisms are well founded; however, allocative decisions within a health care system have to be made, and CUA is the most sophisticated method of economic evaluation so far developed to aid such decisions.

Suggested reading

Bowling A. *Measuring health. A review of quality of life measurement scales.* Buckingham: Open University Press, 1991.

Bowling A. *Measuring disease. A review of disease-specific quality of life measurement scales.* Buckingham: Open University Press, 1995. (Two exhaustive reviews of both generic and disease-specific QOL measures.)

Brooks RG. *Health status measures in a changing world.* London: Macmillan, 1995. (Review and issues about the development and use of QOL measures.)

Cavallo MC, Sassi F, Geraci P. Analisi costo utilità della terapia intensiva nel trattamento dell'ictus emorragico. *Mecosan* 1994:**11**:28–37. (The example in this chapter was based on this study.)

EuroQol Group. EuroQol: a new facility for measurement of health related quality of life. *Health Policy* 1991;**16**:199–208. (Description of the EuroQol instrument.)

Gerard K. Cost–utility in practice. A policy maker's guide to the state of the art. *Health Policy* 1992;**21**:249–9. (Methods used in CUA studies have developed since this review, but it is an important review of the way CUA was applied.)

Hopkins A, cd. *Measures of the quality of life and the uses to which such measures may be put*. Royal College of Physicians of London, 1992. (Reviews and issues about the development and use of QOL measures.)

Jenkinson C, Gray A, Doll H, *et al.* Evaluation of index and profile measures of health status in a randomised controlled trial: comparison of the medical outcomes 36-item Short Form health survey, EuroQol and disease specific measures. *Medical Care* 1997;**35**:1109–18. (Provides data to illustrate why QALY measures based on different health outcome measures might not be comparable.)

Johannesson M, Pliskin JS, Weinstein MC. Are health years equivalents an improvement over quality-adjusted life years? *Med Decision Making* 1993;**13**:281–6.

Kind P, Dolan P, Gudex C, Williams A. Variations in population health status: results from a United Kingdom national questionnaire survey. *BMJ* 1998;**316**:736–41.

Mehrez A, Gafni A. Healthy years equivalents versus quality adjusted life years: in pursuit of progress. *Med Decision Making* 1993;**13**:287–92. (These two papers describe the role and limitations of QALYs and HYEs.)

Petrou S, Malek M, Davey P. The reliability of cost–utility estimates in cost per QALY league tables. *Pharmaco Economics* 1993;**3**:345–53. (A warning that the uncertainty about the measures of cost–utility reduces the validity of rankings of cost–utility of different types of healthcare.)

Rosser RM, Kind P. A scale of valuation of states of illness: is there a social consensus? *Int J Epidem* 1978;**13**:117–23.

Ryan M. Using conjoint analysis to take account of patient preferences and go beyond health outcomes: an application to *in vitro* fertilisation. *Soc Sci Med* 1999;**48**:535–46. (A good example of conjoint analysis.)

Research steps for a cost-utility analysis

Stage of economic evaluation	Example
Specification of the question, and baseline comparison group	Whether patients admitted with stroke should be treated in intensive care units or in medical wards (baseline)
Specification of the viewpoint, type and coverage of economic study	Health care providers and patients
Specification of key outcome and estimation of effectiveness	Survival and quality of life at 6 months, effectiveness estimates based on observational cohorts for admitted cases
Specification of method for valuation of health outcomes	Quality of life expectancy, using Rosser–Watts utilities for health states. Health states from questionnaire to patients or carers
Definition of costs to be estimated	Hospital costs only. Indirect costs assumed not to be difference
Estimation of differences in quantities of resource use	Hospital records
Estimation of unit costs of elements of resource use	Excluded common items of equipment, unit costs based on acquisition costs for drugs and consumables, shadow prices for tests based on market prices. Bed days in ICU and medical ward costed from hospital ward budgets
Specification of analytic model	Simple comparison of difference in costs with difference in quality adjusted life expectancy
Taking account of time preference	Short-term period for follow-up, so not relevant
Summarise economic result	Incremental cost per quality adjusted life expectancy
Sensitivity analysis	Model varying laboratory costs of alternative treatment options

7 Cost-benefit analysis (CBA)

At times it is necessary to take decisions on the allocation of resources of large and far reaching interventions which have costs and consequences for more than one sector of society. We may also have to make decisions about whether an intervention is worth making at all. Health care interventions may be competing for resources with other programmes, not necessarily directly linked to health. The type of economic evaluation which can assist planners and decision-makers on such issues is cost-benefit analysis (CBA), which is the first analytical study design to have been introduced in health economics (its origins date back to the 1930s). CBA has been used to evaluate large public programmes such as the building of the Forth and Tay bridges and, later, the third London Airport, the Channel Tunnel, and Victoria Line on London Underground.

/CBA aims to compare all social costs and consequences across different interventions or against a do-nothing option/ At the basis of CBA is the concept that social welfare exists and can be maximised by moving additional productive resources to aspects of production where there is greater social benefit at the margin. Efficient allocation of resources *within* different sectors of the economy may not necessarily be a socially optimum policy therefore the economist has to assume a societal perspective when carrying out this type of analysis./The key to CBA is the systematic calculation of all costs and consequences accruing to society from different options and the expression of their values in monetary terms/ Such an expression allows comparison of competing and different interventions from different sectors of the public economy and allows decisions to be taken on the basis of different returns from investing in different sectors of the economy. Evaluation designs that we have described up to now value consequences either by assuming them as equivalent (CMA), or in utilities (CUA) or in natural units (CEA), while CBA values them in monetary units. What distinguishes CBA from all other economic studies is the fundamental question that it aims to answer, i.e. is that intervention worth doing at all? In CEA or CMA the health target to be achieved has been already agreed; all that remains to be evaluated is the cheapest way of achieving it.

In CBA a list of the types of resources required for the alternative programmes compared is compiled. The aim of monetary valuation of these resources is to assess the value to society, which is not necessarily reflected in the market price of each resource. This may be either because of "imperfections" in the market for the resource (monopoly power, for example) or because a resource is not traded in the market (volunteer labour, for example)/ CBA, as an explicit listing of all costs and consequences of a particular course of action, is necessary whenever goods such as health care do not have a fully functioning market which assigns them values./As large public schemes involve costs and consequences which go beyond personal preferences which generate market prices, some societal items require valuation through CBA. For example, those that benefit from a vaccination programme against an infectious disease are not just those persons who receive the vaccine, but also those persons born and unborn who benefit from a general reduction in infectivity because their present or future chance or catching the infection is lowered by immunization of others. This, in turn, will result in a higher level of health of current and future generations which can, in turn, lead to improved present and future economic welfare./The adoption of an individual viewpoint would lead economists to consider only the costs and consequences of the vaccine, valued through market prices on the basis of individual preference. Such a viewpoint would not consider all external benefits and costs (known as *externalities*) which would accrue to society as a whole.

Translating health consequences in monetary values is far from easy, and such difficulties have contributed to the relative fall from grace of CBA design. Several approaches to valuation have been used. These fall into two broad categories: *individual* or *societal preference* and *human capital*.

Methods for valuing preferences can be either explicit or implicit. Implicit methods rely on the observation of societal behaviour and the derivation of values from such behaviour. For example, British soldiers' pay is enhanced by the so called "X factor" which is a compensation for the turbulence and risks of service life. Similarly, steeplejacks are paid "danger money" for the risks they take in carrying out their jobs. Such enhancements of pay represent the cost that individuals attach to such increased risks. By comparing such implicit valuations we can derive values of risks to be used in the valuation of consequences. Equally, societal values can be derived by looking at past analogous behaviour in the allocation of resources. Costs then assigned to achieve such consequences can be taken to represent the minimum implicit values of the benefits accrued by those decisions. For instance, Mooney estimates that society valued the life of a child at less than £1000 by analysing the expenditure on child-proof medicine containers.

Such valuations are limited by the finite number of examples available, so that other techniques are required to fill the gaps. Such techniques rely on direct explicit eliciting of individual preferences and are known as contingent valuation (*willingness-to-pay*—WTP, and *willingness-to-accept*—WTA).

WTP relies on the views of samples of the general public who are asked how much they would be prepared to pay to accrue a benefit or to avoid certain events. WTA, conversely, is based on the minimum amount a person or population would have to be paid to accept the loss or reduction of a good or service.

The classic WTP (the most frequently used technique) approach relies on questioning an individual's willingness to pay to diminish the probability of a health state (usually adverse) coming into being.

Contingent valuation (CV) has been used to value:

- preventive technologies (such as devices to lower the risk of injuries in traffic accidents);
- treatment and services (such as a community scheme to visit elderly residents or a reduction in pain following surgery);
- health states (such as people's WTP to be rid of symptoms such as nausea, coughing and so on).

Although theoretically more correct and very useful to answer difficult questions in a range of disciplines, direct CV techniques have several shortcomings which relate mainly to the way in which questions are phrased, the link between social class and respondents' income and their valuations of such health states.

Another limitation of this approach is the unreality introduced by questions such as: "what percentage of annual disposable income would you be prepared to give up every year to diminish the chance by 10% of having a foot amputated?". Approaches that have couched such questions using the analogy of insurance premiums have probably been more popular because respondents are more familiar with such concepts.

/ The human capital (HC) approach to valuation is based on an individual's worth to society calculated on the basis of his or her present and future earnings. Each person represents a productive resource to society and illness diminishes that person's productive capacity, which is usually valued in this approach by his or her loss of earnings. Such an easily understandable concept has been widely used to value life and absence from work due to illness. Life, for instance, has been valued on the basis of its expectancy multiplied by the annual average income of that person or that social class. Loss of life has been valued as the loss of projected earnings from the date of death to the projected date of retirement. The same method has been used to calculate daily productivity losses due to short-term illness. Lives can also be valued using CV, the restitution cost approach (from the judiciary), and the implicit preference method (see above). All of these methods have practical and theoretical limitations; however, in general, HC-based methods have gone slowly out of favour, being replaced by WTP-based approaches. In 1993 the Department of Transport valued an "average" life at about £750 000. This figure and others available in the literature can be used (updated annually by the Retail Price Index) but the results should be subjected to sensitivity analysis.

Any decision about spending implies an expression of time preference. Usually, health care programmes evaluated by CBA extend several years into an uncertain future and have an immediate sizeable effect on resources but long-term effects on health. These types of programme may still have to be compared and their values translated into a single current measure which represents their present value. Such a value is usually calculated by *discounting* their future costs and consequences in time. Discounting takes account of observed economic behaviour which shows a positive preference for benefits now and costs later. Discounting consists of decreasing annual values by a rate, called the discount rate, which (in theory) expresses society's preference and its strength. Discounted benefits and costs are valued less the further into the future they accrue.

It is accepted practice for evaluations to present results using a range of discount rates, including both the current government recommended discount rate for public expenditure programmes and no discounting. This allows the choice and use of a discount rate to be one of the variables in the sensitivity analysis.

The assumption of a societal perspective implies that all those costs which are transferred from one area of society to another (such as VAT on drugs) are discarded. Equally, an effort must be made to identify and separate those resources which may be used jointly by two different programmes which are competing in the analysis, such as joint capital costs, by different programmes which share the use of clinic space.

Finally, in CBA, as in all the designs that we have discussed so far, all inputs and consequences must be measured, valued, and costed to reflect opportunity costs, and all steps of economic practice that have been described so far must be observed.

Scenario for cost-benefit analysis

The policy for preventing acute hepatitis B (HB) in a country with an intermediate level of endemicity is to vaccinate all at-risk groups. As this policy is deemed not to be effective in ensuring high compliance, the government is considering the possibility of introducing mass vaccination. As such a decision would entail a major use of resources, and as other important programmes are competing for those resources, health officials decide to carry out an evaluation of desirability of the programme.

Hepatitis B (HB) is a global acute and chronic hepatic viral disease with an estimated 300 million carriers worldwide. HB carries a heavy disease burden in developing countries and a heavy resource burden in developed countries. As HB virus is involved in the genesis of cirrhosis and primary hepatoma, the advent of a plasma-derived vaccine in the early 1980s, and of a genetically engineered vaccine some years later, was hailed as the first effective vaccination against cancer. Such advances and the undoubted seriousness of the disease have put an onus on governments to consider introducing mass vaccination in preference to the vaccination of high-risk groups such as homosexuals, drug users, and health care workers.

Dr Coombe is a public health physician working in the Ministry of Health of a country with intermediate endemicity of the disease which has an annual incidence of about 7 cases per 100 000 population with wide within-country geographical variation and an apparently spontaneous declining incidence.

A programme to target high-risk groups had been started 5 years before, achieving a good coverage rate for health care workers but a low pick-up rate for the other two groups.

As previous mass vaccination campaigns had obtained very high (98%) coverage rates, the minister was keen to extend HB vaccination cover to all the population as a vehicle for achieving coverage of present and future high-risk groups.

Dr Coombe is given the task of evaluating such an investment within the annual spending round. As other programmes competing for ministry funds are backed up by a full CBA, Dr Coombe decides that the HB programme, too, should be evaluated in this manner and asks the help of the economist in his department, Dr Stones. Dr Stones points out that he has recently read a systematic review of similar evaluations on the same topic which contained a long bibliography with a number of studies reporting good-quality *ad hoc* costing. The review concluded that the evidence for mass vaccination was not clear-cut and differences in methodology made extrapolation of the conclusions unreliable. However, the use of such literature and of the available information in the Ministry is easier and cheaper than undertaking a prospective CBA of HB vaccination. Stones, in other words, suggests constructing an economic model based on available data.

Firstly, they set out to value potential benefits of the vaccination programme. Ideally, a sample representative of the entire population would be interviewed to derive an average societal WTP value to avoid HB. Such a scheme is discarded because of its cost and the objective difficulty in getting reliable answers to a question which assumes knowledge of such a complicated disease. Coombe and Stones then set out to estimate the yearly number of probable cases and to map the quantity of resources for a "typical" case.

From their country's epidemiological literature they calculate the yearly number of cases broken down by age and sex adjusted by 25% for under-notification. Given the declining incidence of HB, Coombe and Stones, on the basis of the advice of their statistician, adopt a model which projects the trend downward 20 years and subsequently holds it steady at a low endemicity level. These cases are, of course, the ones that would arise if the current high-risk coverage strategy were to be continued unchanged ("do-nothing strategy").

Next, they deal with the problem of costing a typical HB case by reviewing current knowledge on the natural history of the disease.

Luckily they manage to retrieve the proceedings of an international conference on HB vaccine which has many good-quality papers on the natural evolution of HB. This, coupled with the results of the systematic review, provide sufficient data to build a rather complicated epidemiological model (see Figure 7.1). The model reflects the clinical progression of HB into acute and chronic phases. The former evolves in months, the latter over several decades. The acute phase is mainly benign but an unknown number of clinical and subclinical cases progress to carrier and/or chronic status. Of these, a proportion eventually die either of liver failure or of hepatoma (primary hepatocellular hepatoma).

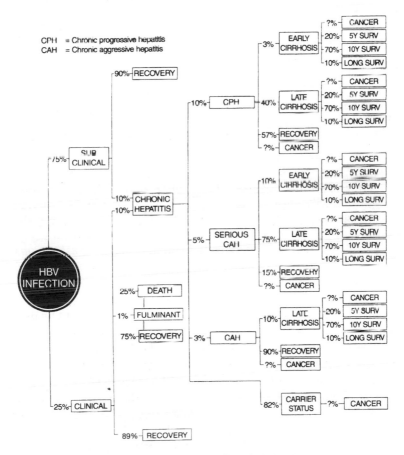

Figure 7.1   *Epidemiological model developed for Dr Coombe's study.*

Coombe and Stones find to their surprise that there is still a degree of uncertainty in the probability of progressing from one form or stage of the infection to another, the relative timespan of each stage, and the likelihood of survival. They load their model on a commercially available electronic spreadsheet and introduce at the beginning of the flow the yearly projected incidence rates, thus deriving yearly numbers of cases for each form of the infection for the following 20 years. Now they proceed to estimate the quantity of resources likely to be used up by each case derived from the model by referring to their available literature augmented by data available in the ministry database. The items they list are:

Direct costs
Hospitalisation
General practitioner time
Diagnostic investigation
Treatment (inpatient and outpatient)

Indirect costs
Tangibles
  Productivity losses, including loss of life (patient and relatives)

Intangibles
  Loss of leisure time (patient and relatives)
  Costs of home help
  Pain, grief and suffering

To calculate hospitalisation rates and length of stay they use national rates specific for each stage of the infection, while they derive GP contacts from similar studies in the literature.

Treatment and diagnostic resource usage they estimate by assuming all treatment as equivalent to the protocols set out by their country's Association of Hepatologists. They also assume complications of cirrhosis to be similar in all forms, i.e. 50% with oesophageal varices, and 50% with all other complications. These assumptions are forced upon them by their inability to find reliable estimates of the incidence of complications.

Productivity losses are derived from the literature, as data on HB-specific absence from work is not routinely collected in their country. The estimates are: 90 days per case for the acute phase, and 180 days per case for all chronic phases. They approximate productivity losses in a family with a minor affected by the disease by assuming that one adult from the family is off work for a period of time equivalent to the length of hospitalisation. Estimates for loss of leisure time (in days) and need for home help are based on a survey carried out a year previously during an epidemic in a representative population.

Hospitalisation costs were from DRG-specific data from one of the regions of the country, while for diagnostic and treatment costs Coombe and Stones use the national tariff. Productivity losses specific to HB infection are unknown, and the only possible alternative is to use national average earnings for those cases which occur during employment. Loss of life due to HB is valued by using a mixed HC-WTP model first calculated by Landefeld and Seskin.

Leisure time was valued by using WTP-based estimates from a previous study, and pain, grief, and suffering by using government figures for compensation of victims of road traffic accidents of various levels of severity.

All costs taken from the literature are updated using the US health care-specific Retail Price Index. To compare like with like, adjustment of cost estimates from different countries and years is needed, because prices of inputs change over time as a result of inflation and differ between countries because of currency differences. There is no perfect method, but theory tells us that inflation adjustment should be based on health care specific price indexes rather than on a more general retail price index, and that conversion between currencies should be based on the purchasing power of the different currencies, rather than on exchange rates which can fluctuate artificially. Purchasing power parity data and health care price indexes are published by the OECD and by the World Bank, but are not always to hand when needed. Fortunately, we and others have found that, although there is a small difference, use of the theoretically less correct retail price index and average exchange rates for conversion of estimates from OECD country studies is not likely to lead to significantly different estimates.

Coombe is somewhat perplexed by what seems to be an exercise based on secondary estimates and average costs. Stones points out that this is the most common type of model and situation to be found in the economic literature of HB. Stones allays Coombe's perplexities by suggesting that average costs are abated considerably during their forthcoming sensitivity analysis and that they adopt a conservative "worst case" position by maximising benefits and minimising costs.

If the programme is still not convenient after such a strategy has been implemented, Coombe may be sure that the intervention is not worth introducing. Coombe realises that economic evaluations, such as the one he has embarked upon, are often used to aid decisions about as yet non-existent services, which is why it is often impossible to collect real data. For this reason, for the costs of the vaccination campaign they include only estimates of the acquisition costs of the vaccine minus VAT, instead of also including costs of storage and cold chain, administration, side effects, surveillance, pain and anxiety, disturbance of families, and publicity of the campaign. They also assume 100% effectiveness of the vaccine.

Their country's recommended discount rate is 8%. This worries Coombe and Stones as it would heavily penalise the many benefits of HB vaccine which would accrue 20 or more years on. They decide to present their results using three different rates, including an 8% rate to see whether the choice of discount rate makes any difference to their conclusions. They lay out their results in a table which looks like Table 7.1.

Table 7.1   Itemised costs by various discount rates of one hepatitis B case (in 1995 US dollars)

| Item | Discount rate | | |
	0%	5%	8%
Hospital	1602	1361	102
GP time	28	23	2
Diagnostic	419	377	45
Treatment	1602	1122	921
Total direct costs	3651	2883	1070
Loss of productivity	4328	2375	1045
Non-marketable (home help)	250	201	71
Pain	385	261	89
Total indirect costs	4963	2837	1205
Grand total of costs	8614	5720	2275

Using average costs in the best-case scenario for vaccination (where benefits and costs are discounted by 0%) benefits equate to costs only after some 35 years. In the worst case (8% discount rate) benefits never reach the level of costs. At this stage it is pointless to continue abating costs to approximate their marginal value as this would only make vaccination even less attractive. To aid their comprehension they present the cumulative curves like those in Figure 7.2.

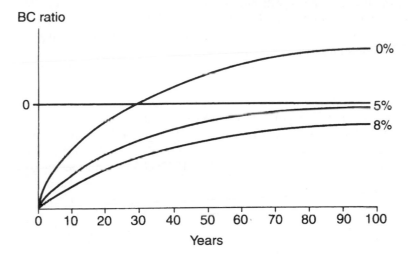

Figure 7.2   *Period of time required for benefits to outweigh costs of HB vaccination by three different discount rates.*

Coombe now suggests using different incidence rates for the infection, assuming a changed under-notification rate. The results show a convenience of vaccination only at incidence levels which Coombe judges unrealistic if compared to current levels of mortality. In other words, mass vaccination is likely to be efficient only at a level of incidence far higher than the present one.

Coombe and Stones conclude that mass vaccination against HB in their country is not a convenient use of resources.

If Coombe and Stones had found that the programme of vaccination would provide a net benefit, they would also have recommended that a formal evaluation be conducted, introducing the programme on a pilot basis at first, to test and confirm or adjust the results of the model.

Readers may be surprised that Coombe and Stones were willing to make decisions on what appeared to be a precarious model with estimates taken from the general literature and numerous epidemiological uncertainties. However, the assumptions they made and the data that were used are not unreasonable and reflect the current state of knowledge, both epidemiological and economic, on the subject. Making allocative decisions has seldom been based on more precise data.

Areas of controversy

Such a powerful technique as CBA has several methodological drawbacks, mainly linked with the crude monetary valuation of complex subjective health consequences as pain, anxiety and death, and estimation of indirect costs.

Three main ethical and methodological objections to the HC approach have been raised (see also Chapter 3).

Firstly, a subject's worth cannot be equated merely to one's productive capacity in paid employment, as such an approach implies that children, the unemployed, the elderly, and the low paid represent low or even negative value to society. This is also a great paradox as those classes of individuals are the ones that are most likely to need health care assistance. Intangible costs (such as pain, grief, and suffering), if valued by HC methods, tend to be small as only the quota which interferes with a person's productive output and costs of therapy and support services is valued.

Secondly, economists dislike the HC approach as it has traditionally tended to overestimate the value of productivity losses by valuing them with average earnings. In a car production line which has 100 workers, if one or two are ill for a few days it is highly unlikely that a high productivity loss for the firm would follow, as the remaining workers would easily cover for the sick. Additionally, in countries of high unemployment, medium to long-term sickness absences would be compensated for by employing out-of-work personnel, hence labour costs, rather than earnings, are a better estimate of productivity losses. Such an overestimation is made worse by the fact that in areas of high unemployment sick workers can often be replaced at little cost to the firm.

Lastly, the HC method carries a risk of counting the loss of productivity and loss of life costs twice, especially when the demarcation between sickness absence and death is unclear.

Such criticisms have led to the introduction of the friction method of valuing productivity losses. The method is based on the empirical observation that real productivity losses to a company are likely to accrue only in the period required to adjust to the new situation created by the sickness episode. After this period (called the friction period) the worker returns from sickness or somebody is hired in his/her place.

Criticism of this concept has centred mainly on the requirement to have an up-to-date picture of the local labour market to be able to estimate the ease of replacement and, hence, the length of the friction period. Such knowledge may not be easy to acquire.

Despite such criticisms, societal economic evaluations of health care programmes require productivity losses, loss of life, and sometimes pain and suffering to be valued.

In our experience, friction methodology or the similar concept of "avoided costs" (see Chapter 3) are a scientifically acceptable alternative to the use of average costs.

The practice of discounting has been subjected to criticism which centres on the right of the current generation to make allocative decisions which will influence generations to come on criteria which include an arbitrary time preference. Discounting is an acceptable practice when making individual choices but is controversial when making societal ones. For instance, the choice of a high discount rate may penalise those programmes in which costs accrue in the first years of implementation and benefits accrue many years into the future—such as a blood-lipid lowering campaign—in favour of other programmes in which both costs and benefits accrue in a short timespan, such as a programme of anti-influenza vaccination.

Suggested reading

Demicheli V, Jefferson TO. Cost-benefit analysis of the introduction of mass vaccination against hepatitis B in Italy. *J Pub Health Med* 1992;4:367–75. (The basis of our example)

Hutton J. Cost-benefit analysis in health care expenditure decision-making. *Health Econ* 1993;1:213–16. (A clear résumé of the rise and fall of CBA in the last 20 years and current prospects for its use with CV-derived estimates.)

Jacobs P, Fassbender K. The measurement of indirect costs in the health economics evaluation literature. *Int J Tech Hlth Care* 1998; **14**: 799–808. (A useful review.)

Jefferson TO, Gray AM, Mugford M, Demicheli V. An exercise on the feasibility of carrying out secondary economic analyses. *Health Econ* 1996;5:155–65. (The paper shows that there is little difference in outcome of secondary economic evaluations between the use of purchasing power parities or a retail price index as a convertor for cost estimates. The exercise was carried out on a model of influenza vaccination.)

Johannesson M. The contingent-valuation method. *Medical Decision Making* 1993;**13**(4):311–12. (A good description of the subject.)

Johannesson M, Jönsson B, Borquist L. Willingness to pay for anti-hypertensive therapy: results of a Swedish pilot study. *J Health Econ* 1991;**10**:461–74. (This is a study comparing different approaches to estimation of willingness to pay for hypertension treatment among 481 patients on an existing hypertension register, currently receiving treatment. The authors compare an open-ended question asking the maximum amount patients would be willing to pay, with a closed set of options to choose an amount out of a given list. A majority could not answer the open-ended question. Some respondents thought they should not have to pay and so would not answer. The closed-ended question resulted in a median willingness to pay of between 2000 and 3000 Swedish kroner.)

Koopmanschap M, van Ineveld M. Towards a new approach for estimating indirect costs of disease. *Soc Sci Med* 1992;**34**:1005–10. (The introduction to the concept of friction period with a critique of HC methodology.)

Landefeld SJ, Seskin EP. The economic value of life: linking theory to practice. *Am J Pub Health* 1982;**72**:555–66. (Contains value-of-life estimates derived from a mixed HC/CV approach.)

Morrison GW, Glydmark M. Appraising the use of contingent valuation. *Health Econ* 1992;**1**:233–43. (A clear review of the rationale for and the use and limitations of CV with a literature review.)

Sheldon TA. Discounting in health care decision-making: time for a change? *J Pub Health Med* 1992;**14**:250–6. (A very clear summary of the rationale and reasons against the practice of discounting, written for non-economists.)

Given the explosion of means of communication such as the world-wide web, and the consequent availability of information, this situation appears a paradox similar to the cry of Coleridge's ancient mariner: "water, water everywhere, nor any drop to drink!" The paradox is more apparent than real. Paper and electronic journals, books and databases, often provide large quantities of unstructured, biased, fragmentary unevaluated and often contradicting information that, if used in a decision-making context, is at best useless and at worst dangerous.

The international scientific community has been aware of this problem for over three decades and, as a result, has developed techniques to assimilate information from different sources in an explicit fashion. One increasingly used method is that of systematic reviewing (see also Chapter 9) and "knowledge-basing" or constructing and maintaining databases of high-quality structured information.

As we have seen in Chapter 5, The Cochrane Database of Systematic Review (CDSR) can help fill some of the gaps. However, reviews contained in CDSR address mainly effectiveness (and sometimes safety) of healthcare interventions. To carry out complex economic evaluations in specific decision-making contexts, additional structured information is needed.

Scenario for economic evaluation and decision-making

The department of a large multinational company that has a workforce with a high rate of absenteeism due to infectious respiratory disease. The Managing Director demands the introduction of measures to prevent the infections and thus minimise their impact. The occupational health staff devise a decision-making model based on the results of workplace health surveillance, the results of three Cochrane reviews, a systematic review of the economics of influenza prevention and an economic evaluation. Lack of effectiveness and concerns over the safety of some of the interventions simplify the decision tree and show influenza vaccination to be a best buy in the case of an impending epidemic.

Mr Long is the Managing Director of a famous large multinational company called "ALD" producing widgets. The company has a multi-ethnic workforce of 100 000 spread over four continents. Three years previously, ALD's chief occupational physician, Dr Spice, had introduced a simple health surveillance system. Dr Spice had devised the system with Mrs Bergperson, ALD's director of nursing services, and called it BS 96 (from the initials of its inventors and the year of its launch). For three years, BS 96 had been producing monthly ICD-based summaries of causes of sickness with their impact on the workforce expressed as working days lost. Spice and Bergperson had always been concerned about the level of morbidity for respiratory diseases but in the last "season" the global picture had got worse.

The aggregate BS 96 returns of the previous twelve months (December 1998 to December 1999) showed that infectious respiratory disease, as defined by history and clinical examination (so-called "clinical definition") had overtaken accidents and injuries and become the highest cause of morbidity and productivity losses (Table 8.1).

Table 8.1   Dr Spice and Mrs Bergperson's BS 96 aggregate returns for clinical respiratory infectious disease in ALD's workforce for the period December 1998 to December 1999. The table shows both the first attendance and any second or subsequent attendance for clinically-defined respiratory disease of a probable infectious nature. Figures are expressed as rates per 100 000 members of the workforce over the year

Attendance	Morbidity	Working days lost
First attendances	620.3	230.8
Subsequent attendances	88.2	16.4
All attendances	804.2	299.7

Dr Spice and Mrs Bergperson decide to present the data to Mr Long during a specially convened meeting. Mr Long's reaction is predictable: "This is very worrying on two accounts. We should look after our people and try and minimise the costs of absenteeism. This is just too expensive to be allowed to continue. Spice, I want you to look at the options and come up with a plan."

Dr Spice and Mrs Bergperson go back to their office and decide to call Dr Dixon (an expert on respiratory disease) to advise them on how to proceed. A week later, Dr Dixon has assessed the evidence provided by BS 96. He suggests that, given that a multitude of agents could be causing the observed respiratory morbidity and that prevention and treatment must be targeted to an agent, a diagnostic survey is required to estimate the burden due to each agent. Dixon suggests that once the survey is finished and the estimates are available, Spice and Bergperson must commission an economic model of competing interventions to look at the "best buy" strategy to comply with Mr Long's directive. Spice and Bergperson now organise a survey based on laboratory isolates and serological antibody titres against respiratory pathogens in a random sample of the workforce reporting sick.

A year later, the survey clearly shows that over the year approximately half of the morbidity is due to influenza A and B, while the rest is due to a variety of agents including RSV, rhinoviruses, adenoviruses and pneumococci. Now Dixon advises Spice and Bergperson to concentrate on devising a decision-making model to prevent and/or treat influenza A and B. The reasons he gives are as follows: "Firstly, the bulk of the yearly morbidity is caused by influenza and that is where we should concentrate to begin with. Secondly, there is likely to be more and better evidence on interventions for influenza than on any of the other agents." Dr Nixon lists the following alternatives to prevent and or treat early influenza in otherwise healthy adults:

- *Vaccines*

  These usually contain a cocktail of antigens of the "current" virus (as the viral configuration changes every year) and are manufactured following a yearly recommendation by WHO.

- *Ion-channel inhibitor antivirals (amantadine and rimantadine)*

  In the USA, amantadine was licensed for the treatment and prophylaxis of influenza A infections by the FDA in 1976 and rimantadine in 1993. In the UK only amantadine is licensed and is administered orally at a recommended does of 100 mg a day in healthy adults for five days (treatment role) or 100 mg a day as long as the risk of infection lasts (prophylaxis role). Both compounds interfere with the replication cycle of type A (but not type B) viruses.

- *Neuraminidase inhibitor (NI) antivirals (zanamivir and oseltamivir)*

  Zanamivir (nebulised) and oseltamivir (taken orally) represent a new class of compounds. Both compounds appear to be effective against influenza A and B, while amantadine is effective only against influenza A.

Dixon insists that the model should be based on the best available evidence of the effectiveness and safety of the various interventions.

Dr Spice consults the Cochrane Library. In the CDSR he finds two reviews on influenza vaccines and ion-channel inhibitors in health adults, but none on NI antivirals. After some discussion, the company offers to finance the production of this review, and the editor of the Cochrane Acute Respiratory Infections Group is able to put Spice in contact with Dr De Vitis, an Italian Cochrane reviewer who would like to carry out the review. De Vitis accepts the task, provided it is supervised by an "at arm's length" steering committee, to maintain scientific independence.

While the Cochrane review is underway, Spice and his team assume a hypothetical scenario in which all available means had a preventive and treatment impact on influenza. They also assume that such means would produce adverse effects and have clinical outcomes not homogeneous for quality of life. In this case, the hypotheses to be tested would be

- choice of the best single alternative;
- choice of the best combination of alternatives;
- choice of the best combination of alternatives depending on the outcome measure considered (avoided cases, quality weighted avoided cases, severity of avoided cases, hospital admissions avoided and working days lost).

They decide to compare these alternatives with the current company policy on influenza prevention (i.e. do-nothing).

Spice and his team draw up a list of questions and possible intervention combinations. At this stage they realise they also require advice from an economist and ask Dr Stones for assistance. Dr Stones is too busy to be able to help, but sends his assistant Miss Newhouse. With the assistance of Miss Newhouse, Spice, Bergperson and Dixon construct a very complicated decision-making tree with 166 terminal nodes. The size of the tree and its sheer complexity are very worrying to the team. However, six months later, when De Vitis' review is ready and they are able to compare the evidence for the three classes of interventions, their task is somewhat simplified as the reviews shed light on some of the effects of the interventions.

Firstly, the interventions are very effective against confirmed influenza A and B (except amantadine and rimantadine which are only effective against influenza A). However, if given to prevent or treat "respiratory illness", i.e. that which is diagnosed clinically, their effectiveness is much lower, calling into question their use.

Secondly, they decide to discard all Cochrane evidence from comparisons based on trials which considered only laboratory-confirmed cases, as the purpose of intervening on the company's workforce is that of diminishing the burden of general respiratory illness. Thirdly, the Spice team is able to discard any interventions for early treatment of influenza as the median gain (0.5 days) is insufficient to justify the use of company funds. Lastly, the Cochrane reviews clearly show that there is currently insufficient evidence of safety and effectiveness for vaccines other than the parenteral ones (i.e. injected), despite encouraging preliminary results for the nebulised variety.

After this preliminary round assessing the evidence, Spice and his team are able to construct a "before and after considering the Cochrane evidence" table of alternatives. This is shown in Table 8.2. At this point, the final criteria for the choice of alternatives are:

- evidence of efficacy;
- evidence of safety;
- practicality of organisational implementation in the setting of the company (getting an international workforce spread in four continents to take regular medication when told to by "head office").

On the basis of the first criterion (effectiveness), all remaining alternatives in the third column of Table 8.2 are practicable and acceptable. However when De Vitis, Spice and Dixon look at the evidence of safety from the Cochrane reviews, they discover that amantadine has an unfavourable safety profile as shown in Table 8.3. The safety profile of rimantadine is slightly more favourable and oseltamivir induces nausea in about 9% of recipients. So, applying the remaining two criteria to the definition of comparators and assuming an average influenza epidemic period of 46 days (as in the trials included in the Cochrane reviews) the alternatives of oral amantadine, oral rimantadine and oral oseltamivir are no longer practicable. It is very unlikely that whole bodies of factory workers would comply with the requirement of protracted daily oral drug schedules.

At this stage, Miss Newhouse suggests confirming this assumption by carrying out a simple time trade-off exercise in which a random sample of the workforce are asked if they prefer the risk of contracting influenza to that of experiencing adverse effects such as nausea or gastrointestinal disturbances.

Table 8.2   Possible alternatives to prevent and treat influenza, before and after reviews of the evidence

Items	Before Cochrane reviews	After Cochrane reviews
Which is the best single alternative for prevention?	Oral vaccines Aerosol vaccines Parenteral vaccines Oral amantadine Oral rimantadine Inhaled zanamivir Oral oseltamivir	Parenteral vaccines Oral amantadine Oral rimantadine Oral oseltamivir
Which is the best single alternative for treatment?	Oral amantadine Oral rimantadine Inhaled zanamivir Oral oseltamivir	None (all compounds shortened duration of illness by 0.5 days)
Which is the best combination of alternatives?	Prevention only Treatment only Prevention treatment	Prevention only
Outcome measure	Laboratory cases Clinical cases Working days lost Hospital admissions Deaths Complications	Laboratory cases Clinical cases
Length of epidemics (i.e. required duration of antiviral and NI antiviral preventive treatment)	84 days (SD = 33.6) according to Communicable Disease Reports *Influenza Surveillance—England and Wales (1991–97)*	62 days (SD = 27) (according to influenza vaccines trials included in the Cochrane review)

Table 8.3   Incidence of adverse effects of amantadine expressed as a percentage of participants

Adverse effect	Amantadine	Placebo	Trials (n)	Participants (n)	Significant
All adverse effects	14.7%	10.4%	6	4274	Yes
Gastrointestinal effects	5.1%	2.4%	5	3336	Yes
Increased CNS	7.5%	4.7%	9	5002	Yes
Decreased CNS	8.6%	7.1%	6	3782	Yes
Skin	1.1%	6.8%	4	918	No

The exercise quickly reveals that healthy adults are unlikely to want to take regular medication that produces undesirable effects in the absence of a direct threat of influenza infection. In Spice's view, two other factors contribute to making the prevention of influenza with antimicrobials and NI antivirals problematic. Firstly, it is doubtful whether the protracted logistical effort involved in maintaining the chemoprophylaxis campaign for 46 days is feasible. Secondly, the level and timeliness of the information required to determine with any certainty the "beginning" and the "end" of the influenza epidemic is unlikely to be available, especially when the workforce is in different areas of the world. The only possible use of oseltamivir that Spice can see at the current level of knowledge is the control of confirmed influenza A and B outbreaks in offices and factories. Such a use would require local diagnostic facilities and swift communication, a system well worth achieving but which at present is not in place.

The only real interventions left considering are vaccines. The highest estimates of vaccine efficacy come from the analyses of vaccines which were shown to match the circulating vaccine strain, following the yearly WHO recommendations. Overall, the vaccine efficacy based on results of the placebo-controlled trials was 37% (95% confidence intervals: 18% to 52%). Expressing the efficacy as a risk difference, on average 7% (95% confidence intervals: 4% to 10%) fewer participants who received matched vaccine suffered influenza like illnesses compared to placebo recipients. The effect of the matched vaccine on serologically confirmed cases was also larger than in any other analysis. Overall, the results of seven trials reporting serologically confirmed cases estimated the vaccine efficacy to be 72% (95% confidence intervals: 54% to 83%). Vaccines are thus very efficacious against influenza A and B.

Sixty-nine percent of recipients of parenteral vaccines in the trials reported local adverse effects (mainly soreness at the site of inoculation).

Now Miss Newhouse points out that the economic evaluation is somewhat simplified as the comparison is only between vaccines and do-nothing. She also reflects that time spent waiting for the production of the Cochrane review on NI antivirals was worth the result as the clarification of alternatives saved the definition of a long and complicated decision-making model. Spice, however reminds Miss Newhouse that he was tasked with presenting the full results of the study to Mr Long, who has been impatiently waiting for them.

Miss Newhouse is willing then to carry out a basic economic evaluation using the simplified decision tree and sets about devising a basic form of CEA and once the preferences are inserted, CUA. Her basic assumptions are in Table 8.4. Using a CEA design, Miss

Table 8.4   Values of variables used in Miss Newhouses's basic evaluation and in the sensitivity analysis

Variable	Basic value	Values in the sensitivity analysis
Population	110 000	110 000
Incidence of influenza	5.7 per 1000	5.7 per 1000–400 per 1000
Effectiveness		
Parenteral inactivated vaccine (denominator size = 6566)	0.21	0.12–0.29% (95% confidence interval for clinical case definition). 0.48–0.79% for laboratory case definition)
Amantadine	0.23	0.11–0.34% (95% confidence interval for clinical case definition). 0.42–0.76% (95% confidence interval for laboratory case definition)
NI antiviral	0.74	0.50–0.87% (95% confidence interval for clinical case definition).0.37–0.65 (95% confidence nterval for laboratory case definition)
Adverse effects		
Vaccine (tenderness)	0.57	0.10–0.57
Antiviral (gastrointestinal)	0.05	0.02–0.05
NI antiviral (nausea)	0.11	0.05–0.11
Individual preferences		
Complete well-being = 1 Nausea and influenza = –0.95	}	25th and 75th percentiles scores of preferences expressed as a combination of category rating and time trade-off
Preventive intervention		
Vaccine unit cost	£3.36(1997)	Not tested
Antiviral unit cost	£0.20 per 100 mg tablet (1998)	Not tested
NI unit cost	£6 (1998)	Not tested
Administration costs for vaccine	Nil	2.9 times vaccine costs
Administration costs for antiviral and NI antiviral	Nil	2 times drug costs
Duration of treatment for antivirals and NI antivirals	62 days	11–122 days

Newhouse's CEA is represented in Table 8.5.

Table 8.5   Results of the cost-effectiveness analysis (cost per avoided case in 1998 £ Sterling by assumption and intervention)

	Vaccine	Amantadine	NI antivirals
Bascline	2807	9458	88193
Effectiveness high	746	2862	75015
Effectiveness low	4912	19777	176387
Maximum duration of NI antivirals and amantadine chemoprophylaxis	2807	18612	173542
Minimum duration of NI antivirals and amantadine chemoprophylaxis	2807	1678	15647
Inclusion of administration costs	8140	18917	176387
Highest incidence	40	135	1257
Highest incidence and highest effectiveness	11	41	1069
Highest incidence and lowest effectiveness	70	282	2514
Highest incidence, highest effectiveness and minimum duration of chemoprophylaxis	11	7	190

The high , basic- and low- effectiveness assumption for the three classes of interventions are equivalent respectively to the upper-, middle- and lower-meta-analytical estimate of effect within the bounds of its 95% confidence intervals. The intervals are contained in the meta-analyses within the three Cochrane reviews.

When Miss Newhouse inserts the individual preferences as weights for the outcomes, all interventions are valued negatively, signifying a negative utility. The workforce sample does not want to run the risk of adverse effects in the absence of a sizeable threat, no matter which intervention is considered.

Now Dr Spicc is able to present the results to Mr Long, but before arranging a meeting, he assembles his whole team to discuss any caveats to be put on his recommendation and any remaining problems. As he glances around the table, he asks members of his study team for their views:

- Dr Dixon feels uneasy at recommending no action; however he agrees that the evidence is compelling and cannot fault the methods used. He urges reappraisal of the issue in the case of an impeding pandemic. Dr Dixon points out that the inclusion of NI antivirals in the model before their licensing and in the presence of little evidence is possibly a little unfair. He too calls for a later reappraisal of their use.

- Mrs Bergperson worries about the logistical burden of arranging anything other than a once-a-year vaccination session for a large global workforce.
- Miss Newhouse states unequivocally that basing her economic evaluation on an overview (i.e. a suite of Cochrane reviews assessing the effects of all interventions to prevent and treat a disease), although quite laborious, simplified the task enormously by defining practical alternatives.
- Dr De Vitis points to the lack of availability of similar overviews of topics in literature. He argues that their ready availability would have saved a lot of work and enabled economists to give a relatively quick answer to the problem. He also feels that the use of the three perspectives was very helpful in clarifying choices.

Dr Spice while agreeing with all his team members says: "At the start of this study, I remember thinking that this was likely to be a clear-cut topic, with plentiful and good quality evidence. Now what are we going to do about preventing respiratory illness caused by the other agents?"

Mr Long once briefed, is astounded at the recommendation and urges Dr Spice to keep the subject under review. He wryly wonders why it has taken so long to advise him to continue doing nothing.

Lessons learnt

The main message of the laborious and convoluted research exercise carried out by Spice and his team is that decision-making based on evidence involves a long search for that evidence, but results can be very rewarding. ALD have saved considerable resources by deciding not to prevent respiratory illness in their workforce at the time. Any effort to do so would have been nugatory.

One of the benefits of insisting on a systematic approach to the collation of evidence is that intervention options are immediately simplified by the demonstration of the impracticality of most of them. Thus incredibly complex decision-making trees can be pruned and simplified with good reason.

A further benefit is the demonstration that no dimension (such as effectiveness or efficiency) has primacy over the others. In the case of amantadine administration to healthy adults, the effectiveness and economics of the compound are irrelevant when compared to its safety, as the compound appears to have serious and relatively frequent adverse effects.

The other side of the coin is represented by the relative lack of universal acceptance by the scientific community of some of the methods used in our example, especially the use of systematic reviews of randomised controlled trials in conjunction with economic evaluations to inform decision-making. Decisions, however must be made and it is reasonable to attempt to make them on the best evidence available.

We have presented an example of a model situation in which a decision was held pending an evaluation, which was specifically designed to inform the decision. The quality, applicability and timeliness, of the evaluation done by Dr Spice and Mrs Bergperson in the scenario we have presented above is not typical of most economic studies that appear in the literature.

The lack of apparent effect of published economic studies on practice has been noticed by several who are concerned about the relevance and importance of economic evaluation research. Studies of the reasons for this have clarified several factors. Economic evaluation studies submitted for publication are seldom performed to inform a specific decision. Indeed, they are often funded by research organisations who are remote from decision-making processes, and conducted by academics with priorities to publish their research rather than to ensure the adoption of their findings. We have already shown that economic evaluation cannot include every factor of importance to decision makers, and that there are different competing interests in the decision-making process. We have also shown that economic evaluation highlights the failure of the real world to meet all the assumptions of economic theory, so it is not surprising if what is loosely termed "psychology" or "politics" should lead to different solutions than are predicted by economic studies.

A final point is that economic evaluation methods, although clearly necessary, are evolving as we write, and it has been shown that the reliability of evidence from them is uncertain. It is therefore not surprising that guides to evidence-based policy making, such as that by Muir Gray, suggest that results of economic evaluations should be used with caution.

Suggested reading

Buxton MJ, Drummond MF, van Hout BA, et al. Modelling in economic evaluation: an unavoidable fact of life. Health Econ 1997;6:217–27. (An easy to read summary of some of the issues.)

Buxton MJ, Hanney S. How can payback from health services research be assessed? J Health Services Res Policy 1996;1(1):35–43. (This paper, based on a series of case studies, illustrates the complexity of the role of evaluation of health technologies in decision making.)

Gray, JA Muir. Evidence-based healthcare. New York: Churchill Livingstone, 1997. (This book illustrates approaches and contexts in which decisions must be made, and although it is slightly dismissive of economic evidence, nevertheless provides a useful insight into where economists should be targeting their work.)

Henshall C, Drummond M. Economic appraisal in the British National Health Service: implications of recent developments. Social Sci Med 1994;38:1615–23. (An investigation into the role of economic evaluation in informing healthcare decisions.)

Hill S, Henry D, Pekarski B, Mitchell A. Economic evaluations of pharmaceuticals: what are reasonable standards for clinical evidence?—the Australian experience. Br J Clin Pharmacol 1997;44:421–5. (A paper which considers the standards of clinical evidence necessary for economic evaluations and draws recommendations based on the Australian experience.)

Jefferson TO, Demicheli V, Deeks JJ, Rivetti D. Prevention and early treatment of influenza in healthy adults. Vaccine 2000;18:957–1000. (The paper upon which the chapter is based.)

9 Current issues

In this chapter we examine some of the issues around economic evaluation which were not mentioned in the methodological parts of the book because their complexity required a basic understanding of the subject matter. As many other topics are currently being debated by economists and researchers, we have picked the ones that we believe are either currently the most important or which are likely to receive the most attention in the future.

The introduction of the 1990 changes in the United Kingdom NHS and the consequent division of the Health Service into policy makers (purchasers) and executive branches (providers) has led to a renewed interest in methods of ascertaining whether interventions work, and in what circumstances (effectiveness), and which offers the best return (efficiency). Subsequent reforms have not altered this emphasis.

This "revival" has led to an increase in the volume of both clinical trials and economic evaluations being carried out and published. An increasing number of trials have an economic component, but overall in the literature they represent probably less than 1%.

We start with a brief overview of whether and how clinical trials should be accompanied by economic evaluations.

As the technique of systematic reviewing (and of its quantitative counterpart, meta-analysis) has rapidly gathered international favour, its economic equivalent has been largely ignored by researchers. As in Chapter 8, we refer to "secondary economic evaluations", i.e. those evaluations which use available data either alongside a review and meta-analysis of clinical trials or as a summary of several self-standing evaluations. The few available attempts at summing-up and synthesising economic data are, however, bedevilled by the overall variable quality of economic literature.

An aspect of the quality of economic literature which has received scant attention is that of its relationship with the process of peer-review. We incorporate a checklist for peer-reviewers of the *British Medical Journal (BMJ)* to assess economic submissions. This checklist will be useful as an aid to getting economic studies ready for submission to major medical journals. The checklist is based on the work of the BMJ Working Party on Guidelines for Peer-reviewing Economic Submissions.

Finally, readers who may wish to pursue an interest in economic evaluation can find an up-to-date list of interest groups whom they may wish to join.

Economic evaluation and clinical trials

Increasingly, clinical trials are regarded as the most powerful tool for assessing the effectiveness of interventions. Purchasers, conscious of their limited resources, aim to favour investment in interventions for which there is reliable evidence of effectiveness. At times, competing interventions show little difference in outcome and little to choose between them. The addition of the economic perspective offers a further dimension of evaluation and helps to illustrate trade-offs in choices for decision-makers. Additionally, prospective economic data collection alongside a trial makes sense and allows the evaluation to be based on reliable estimates of effectiveness.

According to Drummond, trialists should assess the following five fundamental aspects when deciding whether and how to introduce economics alongside a trial.

1. Suitability of the trial

- Economic evaluations should not accompany poorly designed trials. The quality of a trial can be assessed according to: robustness of concealment of allocation, size of the sample, and blinded assessment of outcomes on an intent-to-treat basis.
- Economic importance of the intervention. Trials that benefit from an economic input include those comparing interventions with widely differing costs or resource consequences.
- Practical importance of the intervention when trials are assessing new interventions compared to existing ones, especially if undertaken in typical settings.

- Organisational issues. Economic evaluation may be a major difficulty when running large multi-centre or international trials, because it can impose unacceptable organisational burdens.

2. Choice of economic study design

- Choice depends on the nature of interventions, characteristics of the health problem and the outcomes. For example, when outcomes are clinically equivalent, CMA is the correct study design. However, this is a rare occurrence, CEA and CUA being the most likely designs. Readers should refer to Chapters 5 and 6 for illustrations of these principles.

3. Data collection methods

- Choice of data will depend on the aims of both trial and evaluation, and the range of costs and benefits considered can be very wide ranging from direct costs to those accruing in the widest societal perspective.
- Some data can be collected only while the trial is running (for instance, information on quality of life) while other economic items can be gleaned in a "parallel" exercise from other sources.
- Choice of method should consider both available sources of data and the need for generalising from the trial setting.

4. Economic data analysis

- Issues of time preference, uncertainty and variability relating to estimates of resources and consequences and their valuation should be addressed. Additionally, trialists should assess the transferability of the results of their trial across different settings.

5. Quality of evaluation

- It is incumbent on trialists to consult economists on these issues at the start of the planning phase of the trial to ensure appropriate use of economic evaluation techniques.

Failure to consult economists and statisticians in the early stages of planning of an economic evaluation alongside a trial is probably to blame for the poor quality of execution and reporting of economics alongside trials.

Uses of economic literature

The increase in economic evaluations between 1979 and 1990 (see

99

Figure 1.1) raises the issue of whether we can transfer results from existing evaluations to other settings.

The organisation of large complex "primary" studies (those that use original data collected specifically for the study) may cost a great deal of money. Given that transferring results is probably cheaper than commissioning new studies (especially if data to answer the study question are already available) it is necessary to explore the question of whether we can use what we have already rather than spend a lot of time and money to reach potentially similar conclusions.

In order to be able to transfer results from one existing primary evaluation to another setting we must adopt a population perspective, a bit like treating primary studies on a certain topic as a collection of broadly similar patients.

However, abundant literature may not be enough *per se* to allow us to generalise—for two reasons. Firstly, coverage of specific topics may be uneven, and secondly, the few critical systematic reviews that exist all point to considerable gaps in the overall reliability of methodology used in economic evaluations.

There are several additional factors that can limit the power of generalisation. The essence of generalisation is the capability of comparing like with like. This is already a difficult task in health care, which is, by definition, in continuous change and is delivered in all countries of the world with different geographical, political, cultural, and epidemiological outlooks. These can be so intertwined as to be very difficult to unravel.

As good economics is based on a sound understanding of how resources are used, it is important to know whether there is any difference in the resource use between country or setting A and B. For instance, health care interventions with similar names, and perhaps even similar aims, may use resources in different ways. This is dependent on the general availability of resources, for instance, between a rich and a poor country, and on whether health services are public or private.

Any attempt at generalisation from existing economic evaluations, no matter how well conducted, also faces problems which are linked to the different methodologies used. For example:

- There may be different methods to enumerate, measure, and value resources which lead to differences in estimated outcome.
- Settings of studies may be different, with different local characteristics, such as, for instance, labour markets which could influence the marginal cost of production losses.

- Methods used in the original studies are often not homogeneous, with, for instance, a different understanding of the methodology of CEA. At times the use or otherwise of discounting and marginal analysis and the viewpoint are different.
- Study design or technologies evaluated may have passed their "sell-by date".

Standardisation of economic methodologies is probably the best way to overcome some of the problems identified. Drummond and colleagues have proposed a standardisation checklist. If such a laudable initiative gathers momentum any benefit will be long term. Additionally, any attempt at standardisation of other methodologies provides an avenue to propose simultaneous rationalisation of economic methodology as in the case of overviews of RCTs.

While we wait for these policies to bear fruit we are still left with the question of whether at present we can make better use of available economic literature. Two models may be followed to attempt to use data from evaluations outside their original setting:

- The "price adjustment" approach. This compares the monetary estimates from different studies after adjustment for price level differences between countries and over time to standardise current values. The issue to be considered is whether the method for conversion of money valuation data makes a difference to the conclusions of the analysis. An exercise carried out to test this approach on the economics of influenza suggests that this issue may not be as important as previously thought.
- The "resource costing" approach. This looks at the possibility for deriving data on resource inputs from existing studies, whether designed as economic evaluations or not, and estimating costs and cost-effectiveness from unit cost data specific to a particular setting. This means estimating packages of resources from primary economic evaluations and locally pricing these resources to achieve an analytical outcome answer (such as the upper and lower bounds of influenza vaccination CB ratio). Such a method is applied in each different context and is therefore homogeneous. This approach may be useful in overcoming many of the economic problems of generalisation (for example, labour markets which may vary enormously). In addition, the sensitivity to certain variables of such a model indicates areas where resources are used differently and therefore where we would have most problems in generalising.

In this way we can identify variables which need not be recalculated in a new study. These are the variables (identified by primary sources) to which outcome estimates are insensitive and which are probably robust enough to be included in any secondary analysis.

Before progressing to assess which methods can be applied to attempt to extrapolate or pool results from primary studies we must remind readers that systematic review methods may also be applied at any stage of economic evaluation for the estimation of any one aspect of cost or outcome. In our example of hepatitis B immunisation, Coombe and Stones took data from secondary sources for the evaluation. To ensure that they had used the best available data from these sources, they should have conducted a systematic search for evidence. This approach is advocated in the field of policy analysis by Chelimsky, but has not so far been formally incorporated in economic evaluation methods.

Secondary economic evaluations

In other disciplines there has been a considerable degree of methodological development on the subject of generalisation of results from "primary" studies. The same cannot be said for health economics. So, which approach should we use to investigate the possibility of retrieving, summing-up, and generalising from the available evidence? Turning to social science for inspiration one finds guidance from the methods and thinking expressed in Light and Pillemer's seminal work on taking a rigorous approach to critically summarising available evidence.

The first question that any reviewer must ask is "what is the purpose of my review?". The answer to such a question is likely to dictate the methods employed in reviewing. For example, if we are trying to explore what is known of a particular economic subject we are likely to retrieve the maximum number of studies possible and our criteria for inclusion in the review will be probably quite lax. This is true for broadly aimed reviews such as those gauging the quality of international economic literature on a broad topic, such as cancer, or those aimed, for instance, at ascertaining the decision-making impact of economic evaluations.

However, if we aim to test the hypothesis that something is economically worth doing then we may need to be careful what we include in our review, especially given the uneven quality of economic literature. Consequently, the number of variables that we examine may be smaller than in an exploratory exercise. We use the conditional tense because we are sailing into uncharted waters, as we are not aware of any true generalisation studies carried out in the field of health economics.

A summary of the characteristics of these two different approaches is given in Table 9.1.

Table 9.1   Types of review (after Light and Pillemer)

Characteristics	Hypothesis-testing	Exploratory
Aim	To test hypotheses	Define what is known: generate hypotheses
Quality check	Required if quality is low	No, usually the more the better
Variables collected	Few	Many
Studies used	Usually few	Usually many
Inference flow	Treatment to clinical outcome	Outcome to treatment
Inference testing	Yes, strong	No
Subset split required	No	Yes
Stratification	When outcomes are related to study characteristics	No

If a hypothesis-testing aim is chosen, a quality check is the next step. This has the aim of allowing only valid studies into the overview and can be based on widely accepted criteria for "correct" methods in economic analysis, such as the ones that we have illustrated in the preceding chapters. It is possible that in certain areas of the literature such stringent criteria would leave only few or no studies.

The next step is to propose a possible methodology to sum up what we know on the economics of a particular problem. We should not discount the possibility of carrying out meta-analyses with individual data derived from valid studies. This method may be used to carry out economic evaluations alongside RCTs; however, longitudinal economic studies are very few.

Summing up outcomes (such as cost-benefit ratios) weighted for sample or study size is equally a difficult route at present as most of the ratios are derived from estimates and not population samples.

At present, the only remaining way of achieving our aim may be that of using sensitivity analysis, which is the classic economic method for dealing with variability derived from estimates.

If one attempts an overview of economic literature on a particular topic a series of additional problems is encountered. There may be a considerable degree of publication bias which could "subtract" from the overview a whole sub-population of studies without our knowledge. Although scarce attention has been paid to this topic in economic evaluation literature, there may be at least three different types of such bias:

- Studies which are carried out to justify decisions already taken may have a higher chance of publication if they confirm the validity of the decision, especially if this is in line with current scientific wisdom.
- Studies which are independent may not be published for reasons which are linked to the outcome of the study. The direction of this type of bias may be difficult to predict because it may be dependent on current scientific opinion or interest.
- Studies which have been commissioned to assist a specific decision-making process may not be published. This type of bias is potentially important as these studies may be well conducted and funded. Their omission in any review is likely to weaken the conclusions.

The yield of studies which computerised searches may achieve is limited, as Figure 5.1 demonstrates. Therefore, an exhaustive review to trace the highest number of studies possible should consist of hand searches and other systematic efforts.

At times, attempts have been made to derive resource estimates from systematic reviews of trials, thereby in effect conducting simultaneous secondary evaluations of both the effectiveness and efficiency of interventions. Unfortunately this approach suffers from the drawback that most trialists have not collected resource data prospectively, and secondary economic evaluations have to make do with what is available and, in most cases, this is not enough with which to construct an economic model.

Methods of secondary economic evaluation are in their infancy and there are few reviews or even experiments which contain such methods. Perhaps readers of this book may want to try their hand in further developing these methods.

Quality and peer-review of economic submissions

As we have seen, the quality of available literature is variable. A high quality is desirable for a series of reasons. First of all, economic literature is that which makes explicit proposals for allocation of resources. Given that, as usual, there is an opportunity cost to any allocation, it is unethical to invest in interventions on the basis of flawed economic evaluations. Secondly, bad evaluations in themselves waste funders' and researchers' resources which could be better employed in other ways. Finally, bad methods are an obstacle to generalisation, an activity which will be much needed in the future as the cost of primary studies increases.

The *British Medical Journal* has published a set of guidelines which aim to give researchers the minimum background guidance on how to conduct an evaluation and, equally important, how to check its quality prior to submission. The checklist is in fact the one used by referees of the *British Medical Journal* when checking economic submissions. The checklist is reproduced in this chapter, and readers will find it useful as an aide-mémoire to sound design.

BMJ referees' checklist (also to be used, implicitly, by authors)

Item	Yes	No	Not clear	Not appropriate
Study design				
1 The research question is stated	☐	☐	☐	
2 The economic importance of the research question is stated	☐	☐	☐	
3 The viewpoints of the analysis are clearly stated and justified	☐	☐	☐	
4 The rationale for choosing the alternative programmes or interventions compared is stated	☐	☐	☐	
5 The alternatives being compared are clearly described	☐	☐	☐	
6 The form of economic evaluation used is stated	☐	☐	☐	
7 The choice of form of economic evaluation is justified in relation to the questions addressed	☐	☐	☐	

(continued)

105

BMJ referees' checklist (*continued*)

Item	Yes	No	Not clear	Not appropriate
Data collection				
8 The sources of effectiveness estimates used are stated	☐	☐	☐	
9 Details of the design and results of effectiveness study are given (if based on a single study)	☐	☐	☐	☐
10 Details of the method of synthesis or meta-analysis of estimates are given (if based on an overview of a number of effectiveness studies)	☐	☐	☐	☐
11 The primary outcome measures for the economic evaluation are clearly stated	☐	☐	☐	
12 Methods to value health states and other benefits are stated	☐	☐	☐	☐
13 Details of the subjects from whom valuations were obtained are given	☐	☐	☐	☐
14 Productivity changes (if included) are reported separately	☐	☐	☐	☐
15 The relevance of productivity changes to the study question is discussed	☐	☐	☐	☐
16 Quantities of resources are reported separately from their unit costs	☐	☐	☐	
17 Methods for the estimation of quantities and unit costs are described	☐	☐	☐	
18 Currency and price data are recorded	☐	☐	☐	
19 Details of currency of price adjustments for inflation or currency conversion are given	☐	☐	☐	
20 Details of any model used are given	☐	☐	☐	
21 The choice of model used and the key parameters on which it is based are justified	☐	☐	☐	☐
Analysis and interpretation of results				
22 Time horizon of costs and benefits is stated	☐	☐	☐	
23 The discount rates are stated	☐	☐	☐	☐
24 The choice of rates are justified	☐	☐	☐	☐
25 An explanation is given if costs or benefits are not discounted	☐	☐	☐	☐
26 Details of statistical tests and confidence intervals are given for stochastic data	☐	☐	☐	☐

(*continued*)

BMJ referees' checklist *(continued)*

Item	Yes	No	Not clear	Not appropriate
27 The approach to sensitivity analysis is given	☐	☐	☐	☐
28 The choice of variables for sensitivity analysis is justified	☐	☐	☐	☐
29 The ranges over which the variables are varied are stated	☐	☐	☐	☐
30 Relevant alternatives are compared	☐	☐	☐	
31 Incremental analysis is reported	☐	☐	☐	☐
32 Major outcomes are presented in a disaggregated as well as aggregated form	☐	☐	☐	
33 The answer to the study question is given	☐	☐	☐	
34 Conclusions follow from the data reported	☐	☐	☐	
35 Conclusions are accompanied by the appropriate caveats	☐	☐	☐	

The checklist above is, however, inappropriate for partial evaluations (such as COI studies). These, by the way, appear to form the majority of economic submissions to medical journals and may represent the first tentative steps that some health care workers are taking on the road to more complex studies. Editors have real problems in assessing such submissions as they are outside the mainstream of evaluations.

The *BMJ* has produced the following checklist for incomplete evaluations:

Partial evaluation checklist

Item	Yes	No	Not clear
Study design			
1 The research question is stated	☐	☐	☐
2 The viewpoints(s) of the analysis are clearly stated and justified	☐	☐	☐
Data collection			
3 Quantities of resources are reported separately from their unit costs	☐	☐	☐
4 Methods for the estimation of quantities and unit costs are described	☐	☐	☐
5 Indirect costs (if included) are reported separately from direct costs	☐	☐	☐

(continued)

107

Partial evaluation checklist *(continued)*

Item	Yes	No	Not clear
Analysis and interpretation of results			
6 Time horizon of costs and benefits is stated	☐	☐	☐
7 The answer to the study question is given	☐	☐	☐
8 Conclusions follow from the data reported	☐	☐	☐
9 Conclusions are accompanied by the appropriate caveats	☐	☐	☐

In general, authors should consider carefully where to submit their economic manuscripts. Specialist economics journals usually publish papers of a technical nature as well as economic evaluations, whereas finding a home for a COI study is more difficult as both general and specialist medical journals are unsure as to what these studies represent. There is no straightforward solution to the problem, other than trial (which can be both heart-breaking and time-consuming), but would-be authors should remember their obligation to use sound and acceptable methods. A researcher's "greenness" to the scene is no excuse for sloppy methods.

Interest groups

There are a few groups of health care workers within the United Kingdom who share an interest in health economics. Their composition and entry criteria vary, and readers may consider getting in touch with the contact person to join and to be kept abreast of developments in the field.

Health Economists' Study Group (HESG)

The HESG is probably the oldest (it started in 1972) and most active of the UK-based groups. HESG members meet twice a year for conferences and have an active electronic network. Membership is limited to economists and researchers active in the field and at the time of writing costs £15 per year.

The HESG is administered from the Department of Epidemiology and Public Health, The Medical School, University of Newcastle upon Tyne, NE2 4HH to whom all enquiries should be directed. HESG maintains a discussion list at http://www.mailbase.ac.uk/lists/healthecon-discuss/. The list is open and anyone can join. The list affords easy access to the wealth of knowledge and experience of its members, as the experiences of Miss Newhouse in Chapter 8 demonstrate.

National Health Service local health economics groups

There are several local groups for discussion of health economics issues and problems within the NHS. These include groups in Northern Ireland, Scotland, and the south east of England—for which details are given, as one example.

South East Health Economics Network (SEHEN)

The SEHEN is an informal network for the health professionals and researchers in the Anglia and Oxford Region who are interested in health economics. The network aims to provide a forum for discussion and holds regular meetings with invited speakers. Interested readers should write to SEHEN c/o Economics Group, National Perinatal Epidemiology Unit, Oxford Institute of Health Sciences, Oxford. The email contact is: Stavros.Petrou@perinatal-epidemiology.oxford.ac.uk

Internationally, although several meetings take place, few groups have permanent structures.

International Health Economics Association (iHEA)

The iHEA was formed in 1994 and is an international association of economists. It aims to increase communication among health economists, foster a higher standard of debate in the application of economics to health and assist young researchers at the beginning of their career. Persons interested in the subject who do not wish to become members are also encouraged to participate in the iHEA's activities. Its inaugural conference was held in May 1996, and yearly membership currently costs US$25, which includes a newsletter and listing in the world directory of health economists. For further information you should write to Bill Swan, Associate Director, International Health Economics Association, 3rd Floor, Abramsky Hall, Queen's University, Kingston, Ontario K7L 3N6, Canada. Telephone (613) 545–6000 × 4871. Fax (613) 545–6353. Email address: swanb@post.queensu.ca. Or visit the iHEA's homepage at http://healtheconomics.org including the links section at: http://www.healtheconomics.org/Links/HealthEco.htm

Cochrane Economics Methods Group (CEMG)

Formally registered as a Cochrane entity in 1998, this includes economists and other health professionals and researchers involved in the Cochrane Collaboration. The group aims to develop and disseminate guidance on how best to incorporate economic evaluation into the Cochrane Review process. Those interested in the work of this group should write to The Administrator, Cochrane Economics Methods Group, School of Health Policy and Practice, University of East Anglia, Norwich NR4 7TJ, UK.

The Collège des Economistes de la Santé

The French health economists' association, was created ten years ago to join together the majority of researchers in the field. To join the College, readers should contact: Philippe Ulmann, Secrétaire Général, Collège des Economistes de la Santé LEGOS, Université Paris IX – Dauphine, Place du Mal de Lattre de Tassigny, 75116 Paris, France. Tel. 01–44–05–47–86 (or 01–49–76–80–77). Fax 01–44–05–41–27 (or 01–49–76–80–46). E-mail: ces@dauphine.fr. The College's web page is at: http://www.dauphine.fr/ces/

Suggested reading

Barber J, Thompson SG. Analysis and interpretation of cost data in randomised controlled trials: review of published studies. *BMJ* 1998;**317**:1195–1200.

Demicheli V, Hutton J. Peer review of economic submissions. In: Godlee F, Jefferson T, eds. *Peer review in health sciences*. London: BMJ, 1999.

Drummond MF. *Economic analysis alongside controlled trials. An introduction for clinical researchers*. London: Department of Health, 1994. (An exhaustive introduction to the subject.)

Drummond MF, Jefferson TO, on behalf of the BMJ Economic Evaluation Working Party. Guidelines for authors and peer-reviewers of economic submissions to the *BMJ*. *Br Med J* 1996;**313**:275–83.

Drummond MF, Brandt A, Luce B, Rovira J. Standardising methodologies for economic evaluation in health care. *Int J Technol Assessment Health Care* 1993;**9**:26–36.

Jefferson TO, Mugford M, Gray A, Demicheli V. An exercise on the feasibility of carrying out secondary economic analyses. *Health Econ* 1996:**5**:155–65.

Light RJ, Pillemer DB. Summing up. *The science of reviewing research.* London: Harvard University Press, 1984. (The universal textbook for systematic reviewing of research.)

Luce B, Simpson K. Methods of cost-effectiveness analysis: areas of consensus and debate. *Clin Therapeut* 1995;17:109–25. (The above paper describes many of the areas where the consensus about methods is still debated, and highlight the need for a common sense and "transparent" approach to any analysis.)

Recommended reviews

Adams ME, McCall NT, Gray DT, Orza MJ, Chalmers TC. Economic analysis in randomised controlled trials. *Med Care* 1992;30:231–8.

Brown M, Fintor MA. Cost-effectiveness of breast cancer screening: preliminary results of a systematic review of the literature. *Breast Cancer Res Treat* 1993;25:113–18.

Cairns J, Shackley P. Sometimes sensitive, seldom specific: a review of the economics of screening. *Health Econ* 1993;2:43–53.

Cohen DR, Fowler GH. Economic implications of smoking cessation therapies. *PharmacoEconomics* 1993;4:331–44.

Daly E, Roche M, Barlow D, Gray A, McPherson K, Vessey M. HRT: an economic analysis of benefits, risks and costs. *Br Med Bull* 1992;48:368–400.

Demichell V, Jefferson TO. An exploratory review of the economics of recombinant vaccines against hepatitis B (HB). In: Ronchi E (ed.) *Biotechnology and medical innovation: socio-economic assessment of the technology, the potential and the products.* Paris: OECD, 1997. pp. 105–23.

Fraser NM, Clarke PR. Cost-effectiveness of breast cancer screening. *Breast* 1992;1:169–72.

Gerard K. Cost-utility in practice: a policy maker's guide to the state of the art. *Health Policy* 1992;21:249–79.

Jefferson TO, Demicheli V. The socioeconomics of influenza. In: Nicholson, Hay and Webster, eds. *Textbook of influenza*, pp. 541–7. London: Blackwell, 1998.

Jefferson TO, Demicheli V. Is vaccination against hepatitis B efficient? A review of world literature. *Health Econ* 1994;3:25–38.

Jefferson TO, Drummond MF, Smith R, *et al.* Evaluating the *BMJ* guidelines on economic submissions – prospective audit of economic submissions to the *BMJ* and *Lancet. JAMA* 1998;280:275–77.

Johannesson M, Jönsson B. A review of cost-effectiveness analyses of hypertension treatment. *PharmacoEconomics* 1992;1:250–64.

111

Udvarhelyi S, Colditz GA, Rai A, Epstein AM. Cost-effectiveness and cost-benefit analyses in the medical literature. Are methods being used correctly? *Ann Intern Med* 1992;**116**:238–44.

Appendix 1: Costing methodology for any type of economic evaluation

Many methodological papers have been published on the subject of cost measurement for health economic studies, and we list some here which are relevant to all the previous chapters.

Further reading

Finkler SA. The distinction between costs and charges. *Ann Intern Med* 1982;**96**:102–9. (An article illustrating the importance of interpreting carefully studies reporting "costs" based on prices charged for health care.)

Finkler SA, Knickman JR, Hendrickson G *et al*. A comparison of work-sampling and time and motion techniques for studies in health services research. *Health Serv Res* 1993;**28**(5):577–97. (Illustrates how more complex methods of measurement do not necessarily improve estimates of resource input.)

Luce BR, Manning WG, Siegel JE, Lipscomb J. Estimating costs in cost-effectiveness analysis. In: Gold MR, Siegel JE, Russell LB, Weinstein MC, eds *Cost-effectiveness in health and medicine*. Oxford: Oxford University Press, 1996. (This is a chapter in a book reporting the consensus of a US Public Health Service task force on methods and principles for economic evaluation.)

Netten A, Beecham J. *Costing community care*. PSSRU Canterbury: University of Kent, 1993. (This paper discusses methods and approaches for aspects of cost where routine data are not usually available and are therefore neglected in most evaluations of alternative forms of care, which become hospital dominated and rather narrow in viewpoint.)

Smith K, Wright K. Informal care and economic appraisal: a discussion of possible methodological approaches. *Health Econ* 1994;**3**:137–48.

Whynes DK, Walker AR. On approximations in treatment costing. *Health Econ* 1995;**4**:31–9.

Simple more aggregated methods of cost estimation may provide unbiased estimates of the more detailed analysis of patient costs. This illustrates the need to consider how much work is needed for cost estimation.

Sources of cost data for the United Kingdom

The Personal Social Services Research Unit (PSSRU) at the University of Kent runs a programme, funded by the Department of Health, which collects and disseminates data on the unit costs of health and social services. The PSSRU produces an annual report which contains up-to-date cost information as well as highlighting recent research work on the subject of costing services.

Reports are available from Anne Walker, PSSRU, The University, Canterbury, Kent CT2 7NF. Website: http://speke.ukc.ac.uk./pssru/publications./html

Information on expenditure by programme in England is available from FCIA-FAST, NHS Executive, Room IN33A, Quarry House, Quarry Hill, Leeds LS2 7UE. *The NHS costing manual* (for finance officers) and *NHS reference costs* are published on the NHS executive web site at http://www.doh.gov.uk/dhhome.htm. Data on hospital and community expenditure broken down by specialty are available from FCIB-FMU, NHS Executive, Room 7N33D, Quarry House, Quarry Hill, Leeds LS2 7UE.

Data on costs in Northern Ireland are available from the Policy and Accounting Unit, Financial Management Directorate, Department of Health and Social Services, Dundonald House, Stormont Estate, Belfast BT4 3SF.

Cost and expenditure data in the Scottish NHS are available from Economics and Information Division, Scottish Office, Room 252, St Andrews House, Edinburgh EH1 3DE.

General background information on costs falling on families is available from HMSO publications such as the *Family Expenditure Survey*.

Appendix 2: Economic logic applied to management of health services—forms of economic appraisal

Economic logic underlies some of the other objects of health economics (see Chapter 1). In the specific case of the management of health services, its application forms the conceptual basis for a set of techniques which have recently gained in favour as tools to manage resource allocation in health services. This appendix will give a brief overview of such techniques and their application. Readers will find examples of their practical applications in the bibliography section. The techniques are:

Programme budgeting (PB), which is a description of the distribution of resources across and within different programmes.
Marginal analysis (MA), which examines the effect of small changes in the existing pattern of health care expenditure in any setting.
Opinion appraisal (OA), which is the systematic examination of the relative advantages and disadvantages of alternative options in meeting specific health objectives before resources are committed to one or more programmes.

In general, PB is frequently used as a descriptive preliminary to MA in circumstances where either little is known about the service (and hence there is a requirement to describe before carrying out an analysis) or where the service is diverse or managerially fragmented (such as in the case of reproductive medicine services). PB is carried out by defining and identifying the programme or programmes in question and then compiling a statement (often in tabular format) of activity and expenditure which is usually known as the "programme budget".

MA usually is carried out from this step onwards. Its nub is the decision of which services are candidates for an increase in resourcing and which for a compensating reduction. Such a decision is usually made through consultation rounds with representatives of interested parties. The next step is that of measuring the costs and consequences of such changes and, once decisions are made, measuring the effect of the changes. Given its rationing ethos, the success of MA relies very much on its acceptance by the population and the media, and consultation is a vital phase of the process.

Because of their sequential logic, PB and MA are often carried out one after the other, and the process is called PBMA.

OA is a tool for strategic resource allocation which consists of four basic steps:

- Stating the strategic planning context.
- Setting the objectives and constraints.
- Formulating options.
- Evaluating options.

In OA, consequences are valued in monetary and in non-monetary terms and, as such, it is an aid to both strategic planning and capital investment programmes.

All three techniques are seen by economists as an alternative to the "classic" epidemiological needs assessment, which is based on a descriptive approach to disease and its impact on society. PBMA and OA can be used for priority setting and the explicit choices which form their basis clearly illustrate the trade-offs imposed by the scarcity of resources.

Suggested reading

Cohen D. Marginal analysis in practice: an alternative to needs assessment for contracting health care. *BMJ* 1994;**309**:781–5.

Department of Health and Social Security. *Option appraisal. A guide to the National Health Service.* London: HMSO, 1987. (A clear step-by-step guide to OA.)

Donaldson C. Economics, public health and health care purchasing: reinventing the wheel? *Health Policy* 1995;**33**:79–90. (This paper sets out the rationale for and the methods of PBMA.)

Henderson J. *Appraising options.* Series of Option Appraisal Papers No. 2. Available from the Health Economics Research Unit, University Medical Buildings, Foresterhill, Aberdeen AB9 2ZD. (A clear step-by-step guide to OA.)

Torgerson DJ, Spencer A. Marginal costs and benefits. *BMJ* 1996;**312**:35–6. (This and the above paper by Cohen are very good examples of the practical applications of marginal analysis.)

Twaddle S, Walker A. Programme budgeting and marginal analysis: application within programmes to assist purchasing in Greater Glasgow Health Board. *Health Policy* 1995;**33**:91–106. (A practical example of PBMA in action.)

Appendix 3: An introduction to health care decision analysis

Background

Health care workers at times are called upon to make decisions which do not involve either risks or uncertainty. Often, however, the facts are far from clear and mistakes affecting either the collection or interpretation of data may have been made, leading to wrong decisions being taken, negatively affecting the lives of patients. A method for decreasing the likelihood of mistakes, and for clarifying a problem, is that of *decision analysis*. Decision analysis is a process which allows us to:

- break a difficult problem down into simpler, more manageable components;
- examine in detail each component part;
- combine each component in a logical sequence to allow us to recognise the best solution.

Probabilities and wagers

Many decision-making problems are similar to wagers. Let us examine the example of a doctor and his or her patient considering whether to undergo either a standard surgical procedure which carries a known success rate and a certain rate of death by complications, or a new procedure which could have a higher cure or success rate but which entails a certain probability of a permanent sequela such as an ugly scar.

The choice of procedure will be very much dictated by the probabilities of the various outcomes (cure, death, and permanent disability rates) and by the values given by the patient to the various possible outcomes (expressed as preferences).

In health care it is often possible to gauge such risks, but this assessment usually carries with it costs such as that of delaying treatment. Additionally, such decisions can be extremely complicated when there are multiple possible outcomes and when patients' values vary one from the other.

Gamblers are successful when they are able to calculate the probability of winning and combine it with possible jackpots. Similarly, doctors and other health care workers can combine risks with patients' preferences.

Decision analysis is an explicit, quantitative and descriptive method as it forces each decision maker to clarify how problems are analysed and how single components are combined when taking the decision. As such, it can be an important aid to decision-making, as the decision maker is obliged to measure or "size" possible alternatives by assigning numeric values both to probabilities and to the outcome of each possible decision. There are five basic steps in decision analysis:

- problem identification;
- structuring the problem and constructing a time horizon;
- measurement of uncertainties (probabilities and utilities);
- uncertainty assessment and choice of the best solution;
- sensitivity analysis.

Problem identification

Carrying on with our previous example, we need to identify all the different treatment options and list them next to each possible length and quality of life outcome. In our case let us assume that these are:

standard treatment: *cure*
> *death*

new treatment: *cure*
> *death*
> *permanent disability* (for example, a scar)

Problem structuring

This is usually done by the use of a decision tree (Figure A1), a flow diagram in which decisions and outcomes are shown in time sequence: early events on the left and later events on the right. Each tree has three types of node:

- decision nodes, shown as squares;
- chance nodes, shown as circles;
- terminal nodes, which are the end of each branch.

There are two basic rules when constructing a decision tree. Firstly, the branches which sprout from a node must be exhaustive and mutually exclusive, and secondly, the sum of probabilities in each branch must be equal to 1.

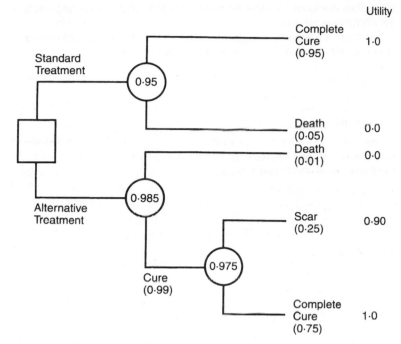

Figure A.1   *Example of a decision tree*

Measurement of uncertainties

Let us assume that we had reliable probability estimates for treatment in our example as follows:

standard treatment: *cure* 0.95
               death 0.5

new treatment: *cure* 0.99
           death 0.1
           scar 0.25 in cured patients

It is now necessary to calculate the utilities attached to the various outcomes of our decisions in order to combine them with each probability and ascertain which decision will yield the most utility. The method frequently used to calculate utilities is that of standardising wagers. The patient is asked to list in order of preference the three possible outcomes (cure, cure with a scar, and death). The patient is likely to assign the highest utility to cure (utility = 1) and the least utility to death (utility = 0). Cure with a scar will probably attract an intermediate utility value. However, to assess the exact utility of the scar outcome we must formulate a series of wagers between immediate death and the scar outcome until the same utilities are reached. This is done as follows.

The patient is asked to imagine being in front of two doors, and that he or she must decide which one to go through assuming that:

- going through the left hand door there is no risk of death but a certainty of an outcome with a scar;
- going through the right hand door there is a 0.50 chance of complete cure but also a 0.50 chance of death.

The patient will probably choose the left hand door. At this point the wager is reformulated, progressively decreasing the risk of death beyond the right hand door up to the point where the patient has difficulty in choosing a door.

Let us now assume that this point corresponds to a risk of death of 0.10 and of complete cure of 0.90. This is the so-called "level of indifference".

There are alternative methods to calculate utility values; for instance, the patient can be asked to assign utility values to the various outcomes on an analogue scale marked 0 to 1. One such method is that of expressing time preferences—for example, asking a patient with a laryngeal carcinoma to trade-off survival time against a period in possession of his or her vocal function. One of the drawbacks of these methods is that patients tend to avoid the extreme values of the scale, whereas other methods which convert utilities into monetary values, or years of life, do not provide linear values (i.e. 0 to 1). Additionally, patients tend to be "risk averse", i.e. future years of life gained are valued less than years to be gained now. These drawbacks make these methods unsuitable for use in decision analysis.

Choosing the best solution

Once utilities are calculated, the next step is to insert them in the model to allow us to choose the best solution. Initially this is done by calculating the utilities in each chance node through the means of a weighted mean of utilities of all possible outcomes in which the weights are given by the probabilities of each outcome. For instance, following Figure A1, the probabilities in the lower (alternative treatment) node are $(1 \times 0.75) + (0.90 \times 0.25) = 0.975$.

When there are several nodes positioned sequentially, as in Figure A1, traditionally the weighted utility of the end node is used to calculate the expected utility of the proximal node. In our example the overall utility of the alternative treatment node is $(0.975 \times 0.99) + (0 \times 0.01) = 0.965$.

The utility attached to a decision node is traditionally assigned as equal to that of its branch with the highest utility. This rule is based on the assumption that any rational decision-maker would choose the solution with the highest utility attached to it. In our example the expected utility for the alternative treatment (0.965) is higher than that of the standard treatment, so that the alternative treatment is most likely to be chosen.

120

The difference in expected utility between the two alternatives could appear as minimal. We must, however, bear in mind that on such a scale a difference of 0.015 is equivalent to 1.5% of the value given to a full and healthy life. Additionally, if our hypothetical patient agrees with the principles of utility theory, and if the probabilities used in our model are the best available, a decision to follow the least-utility strategy would be perverse (regardless of the minimal difference involved).

Sensitivity analysis

The final stage is that of sensitivity analysis, which must be undertaken given the uncertainty which, in practice, surrounds the utilities and probabilities used in decision analysis. In a sensitivity analysis each probability and utility estimate is sequentially varied within a reasonable confidence interval to test the robustness of the conclusions reached.

In our example the utilities attached to the two treatments are equivalent for a scar outcome utility estimate of 0.85. Beyond this value the alternative treatment becomes more attractive than the standard one. The point of equivalence is called a "decision threshold". This threshold varies as the estimates of other variables are changed. The structure of decision trees and the high number of variables to be tested in a sensitivity analysis can often engender problems which, unlike our simple example, can be handled only with the help of a computer programme.

Conclusions

Decision analysis is rarely used in planning the treatment of single patients. Up to now its applications have been limited to aiding the debate on treatment of whole categories of patients or conditions for which there is considerable uncertainty or controversy. However, decision analysis techniques have many useful applications in, for example, the field of clinical trials or public health as a framework for resource allocation decisions based on economic principles.

In conclusion, decision analysis forces the operator to examine a problem in a systematic manner and to value its components explicitly. It also helps to manage complex problems and to limit mistakes. Its main drawbacks are its time-consuming nature and potentially complicated nature which, at times, makes it difficult to explain or teach.

Suggested reading

The following is a selection of easy-to-follow and not-so-easy-to-follow articles and textbooks on decision analysis.

Hillner BE, Smith TJ. Efficacy and cost effectiveness of adjuvant chemotherapy in women with node-negative breast cancer. *N Engl J Med* 1991;**234**:160–8.

Knill-Jones R. Medical decision making in the 1990s. *Theor Surg* 1990;**5**:137–40.

Lilford RJ. Trade-off between gestational age and miscarriage risk of prenatal testing: does it vary according to genetic risk? *Lancet* 1990;**336**:1303–5.

Lilford RJ, Thornton J. Decision logic in medical practice. *J R Coll Physicians* 1992;**26**:400–12.

Llewellyn-Thomas HA, Sutherland HJ, Thiel EC. Do patients' evaluation of a future health state change when they actually enter that state. *Med Care* 1993;**31**:1002–12.

Luce BR, Elixhauser A. Decision analysis. In: Luce BR, Elixhauser A, eds. *Standards for the socioeconomic evaluation of health care services*. Berlin: Springer-Verlag, 1990:117–23.

Pauker SP, Pauker SG. Prenatal diagnosis: a directive approach to genetic counselling using decision analysis. *Yale J Biol Med* 1977;**50**:275–89.

Richardson DK, Gabbe SG, Wind Y. Decision analysis of high-risk patient referral. *Obstet Gynaecol* 1984;**63**:496–501.

Weinstein MC, Fineberg HV. *Clinical decision analysis*. Philadelphia: WB Saunders Company, 1980.

Appendix 4: Glossary

Conjoint analysis A technique originally developed in market research aimed at establishing the relative importance of different attributes in the provision of a good or a service and used to estimate how individuals trade between these attributes. If cost is included as an attribute, the technique allows the calculation of the willingness to pay.

Consequence In this book, "consequence" means any change in the natural history of a disease or diseases brought about by interventions.

Contingent valuation (CV) One of the approaches to valuation of costs. The term comprises willingness-to-pay and willingness-to-accept techniques.

Cost The value of opportunities lost by engaging resources in a service (also known as *opportunity cost*). Usually quantified by considering the benefit accruing by investing the same resources in the best alternative manner. The concept of opportunity cost, which is at the heart of economics, derives from the notion of scarcity of resources. Taking the production process into consideration, costs may be differentiated as follows:

Average costs These are equivalent to the average cost per unit. They equate to the total costs divided by units of production.

Fixed costs Those that, within a short timespan, do not vary with the quantity of production—for example, overheads for heating and lighting of a building.

Incremental costs The difference between marginal costs of alternative interventions.

Marginal costs The cost of producing an extra unit of a service.

Total costs All costs incurred in the production of a set quantity of service.

Variable costs Those that vary with the level of production and are proportional to quantities produced.

Taking health problems into consideration, costs may be differentiated as follows:

Avoided costs   Costs caused by a health problem or illness which are avoided by a health care intervention. Estimation of avoided costs is one of the ways of assessing the value of benefits of health care intervention. Sometimes known as benefits.

Direct costs   Those borne by the health care system, community and patients' families in addressing the illness (for example, diagnosis or treatment costs).

Indirect tangible costs   These are mainly productivity losses caused by the problem or diseases, borne by the individual, family, society, or by the employer.

Indirect (intangible) costs   These are usually the costs of pain, grief, and suffering, and the loss of leisure time. The cost of a life is usually included in case of death.

Cost-benefit analysis (CBA)   A type of economic study design in which both inputs and consequences of different interventions are expressed in monetary units. This allows their direct comparison across programmes, even outside health care.

Cost-effectiveness analysis (CEA)   A form of economic study design in which consequences of different interventions may vary but can be measured in identical natural units; relative inputs are then costed. Competing interventions are compared in terms of cost per unit of consequence.

Cost-minimisation analysis (CMA)   An economic study design in which consequences of competing interventions are the same and in which only inputs are taken into consideration. The aim is to decide the cheapest way of achieving the same outcome.

Cost-utility analysis (CUA)   A form of economic study design in which interventions which produce different consequences in terms of both quantity and quality of life are expressed as utilities. These are measures which comprise both length of life and subjective levels of well-being (the best known utility measure is the quality-adjusted-life-years or QALYs). In this case, competing interventions are compared in terms of cost per utility (cost-per-QALY).

Discounting   A technique which allows the calculation of present values of inputs and benefits which accrue in the future. Discounting is based mainly on a time preference which assumes that individuals prefer to forego a part of the benefits if they accrue it now, rather than fully in the uncertain future. The strength of this preference is expressed by the discount rate which is inserted in economic evaluations. The choice of a discount rate, and to which items it should be applied, are a matter of intense debate among economists.

Economic evaluation   The application of analytical methods to define cost and consequences of interventions and aid explicit choice-making in resource allocation.

Efficiency   Making the best use of available resources. The two types are:

Allocative efficiency, which assesses competing programmes and judges the extent to which they meet objectives.

Technical efficiency, which assesses the best way of achieving a given objective (also known as X efficiency).

Equity   Fair distribution of resources or benefits.

Externalities   These are negative or positive utilities accruing to an individual from another person's consumption. For example, if the majority of a community is vaccinated against an infectious disease, the resulting herd immunity benefits those who have not been vaccinated.

Human capital   A method of valuation which equates the value of a person with his or her lifetime earning capacity.

Marginal analysis (MA)   The process which examines the effect of small changes in the existing pattern of health care expenditure in any setting.

Marginal benefit   The value of benefit deriving from an extra unit produced.

Option appraisal (OA)   The systematic examination of the relative advantages and disadvantages of alternative options in meeting specific health objectives before resources are committed to one or more programmes.

Price   Price reflects the value of resources for which there are markets.

Productivity losses   (see also indirect costs) The value of production output loss through morbidity or morality.

Programme budgeting (PB)   A description of the distribution of resources across and within different programmes.

Resources   Classically, land, labour, and capital. Specifically, any input into health service production (time, goods, equipment, buildings, specialised knowledge, etc).

Sensitivity analysis   A technique which repeat the comparison between inputs and consequences, varying the assumptions underlying the estimates. In so doing, sensitivity analysis tests the robustness of the conclusions by varying the items around which there is uncertainty.

Standard gamble   See "Time trade-off", below.

Time trade-off   This (and standard gamble) are valuation techniques based on eliciting preferences for a set health state or a set time given a certain probability of that event happening.

Utility   A term used by economists to signify the satisfaction accruing to a person from the consumption of a good or service. This concept is applied in health care to mean the individual's valuation of their state of well-being deriving from the use of health care interventions.

Willingness-to-pay (WTP) A technique which relies on direct explicit eliciting of individual preferences in the views of samples of the general public who are asked how much they would be prepared to pay to accrue a benefit or to avoid certain events.

X efficiency See "Technical efficiency", under "Efficiency".

Index